www.ingramcontent.com/pod-product-compliance
Lightning Source LLC
LaVergne TN
LVHW012356270326
835020LV00049B/1344
9781068219368

COGNITIV
E
PROCESSI
NG
THERAPY
FOR PTSD

Practical Strategies for Effective

Trauma Recovery

Dr. Christine Herman

COGNITIV
E
PROCESSI
NG
THERAPY
FOR PTSD

Practical Strategies for Effective Trauma Recovery

Dr. Christine Herman

CONTENTS

INTRODUCTION

In today's fast-paced world, where the demands on healthcare providers and mental health professionals are ever-increasing, finding time to reflect, recharge, and rejuvenate can often seem like a distant dream. This book serves as both a guide and a companion to help reclaim that valuable time, offering a deep dive into the intricacies of trauma therapy through the lens of Cognitive Processing Therapy (CPT). It's crafted with you in mind—healthcare providers, researchers, clinical supervisors, educators, graduate students, trainees, and mental health professionals—each seeking to understand better and address the complex realities of mental health and trauma.

Trauma is a profound element of human experience, affecting individuals in myriad ways that ripple through their personal and professional lives. As such, understanding and treating trauma requires not only empathy and insight but also a structured approach grounded in scientific inquiry. This book offers a comprehensive exploration of the principles of CPT, and by doing so, aims to empower you to face trauma confidently and compassionately.

CPT, an established therapeutic modality, offers a framework designed to understand and alleviate the psychological burdens carried by those suffering from trauma-related disorders. It's rooted in the understanding of how cognitive processes are altered by trauma and provides evidence- based strategies to address these changes effectively. In the chapters that follow, you'll journey through the essential components of CPT, encompassing everything from understanding core symptoms to building therapeutic alliances that foster healing and resilience.

Starting with the fundamentals of PTSD, we set the stage to elucidate the nature of trauma and its pervasive impacts on day-to-day life. It's crucial to appreciate how deeply PTSD can integrate into one's existence before effectively facilitating change. Through exploration and understanding of these elements, therapists can create meaningful connections and offer strategic interventions that genuinely resonate with their clients.

The path to transforming trauma involves not just understanding individual experiences but also recognizing the influence of cultural, societal, and familial contexts. This book emphasizes the importance of adapting and tailoring therapeutic techniques to meet the diverse needs of each client. It's not just about following a structured protocol; it's about integrating sensitivity and adaptability into your practice.

The nuances of trauma therapy call for a delicate balance—being both guided and guiding. As professionals, maintaining this balance is imperative to navigating the therapeutic process successfully. Each chapter of this book builds on the last, equipping you with the skills necessary to enhance your therapeutic efficacy and ensure that you are continually evolving in your professional journey.

As you delve into the essence of CPT, you'll engage with methods of identifying and challenging maladaptive thought patterns, teaching emotional processing, and helping clients to construct and navigate their trauma narratives. These techniques are crafted to not only support the individual's healing but also to fortify you as a practitioner, ensuring your strategies remain both effective and compassionate.

While the techniques discussed herein are fundamental to the structure of CPT, no two therapeutic journeys are the same. This book encourages you to explore ways of harmonizing these structured approaches with your personal therapeutic style and intuition, allowing for a more deeply personalized approach to care.

In this way, trauma therapy becomes more than just a professional obligation; it transforms into a dance of self-discovery and growth for both you and your clients. The discussions on diverse populations, safety planning, and dealing with special considerations further enhance your ability to accommodate and adapt to every unique therapeutic encounter.

Equally important to understanding the client's journey is recognizing the trials faced by therapists themselves. This book dives into navigating therapist challenges, overcoming barriers to treatment, and the crucial aspects of professional support and supervision. Providing such reflective insights aims to nurture your professional journey and help you stay attuned to your own needs and the transformations you facilitate.

In the evolving landscape of therapy, exploring new frontiers like technology's role in CPT delivery and long-term management strategies ensures that your practice remains on the cutting edge, enhancing both accessibility and effectiveness. As the therapeutic field continues to advance, opportunities for continuing education become ever more critical. This text thus offers a roadmap to ongoing learning and collaboration, promoting innovation in trauma therapy practices.

Ultimately, the quest to reclaim time and mental space is a shared journey. As you engage with this book, draw upon the collective wisdom it offers

—knowledge that has been gathered through years of clinical practice and research. Let it guide you and inspire you to make profound impacts in the lives of those you serve, and in your own life.

May this book not only serve as an educational resource but also as a source of motivation. Remembering that in choosing to understand and work with the complexities of trauma, you are part of a broader movement toward healing and hope. As you turn the pages, let them unveil the possibilities that lie ahead, both for your clients and for yourself. Together, let's embark on this transformative journey towards greater understanding, resilience, and empowerment.

CHAPTER 1

UNDERSTANDING PTSD

Trauma leaves an indelible mark, reshaping the landscapes of the mind and spirit. As health care providers, researchers, clinical supervisors, educators, graduate students, trainees, and mental health professionals, it's crucial to comprehend the nuances of PTSD to effectively guide the healing journey. Understanding PTSD means recognizing its multifaceted nature, where symptoms like intrusive memories, avoidance, and hyperarousal intertwine in a complex dance that demands both empathy and expertise. The diagnosis criteria offer a roadmap, yet each patient's experience is unique, often impacting daily life in profound ways. By delving into these intricacies, we can cultivate a deeper connection with those we aim to help, ensuring our approaches are not only evidence- based but also infused with compassion. This understanding empowers us to reclaim time and mental space for our patients and ourselves, paving the way for recovery and resilience.

Trauma's effects reach far beyond immediate physical injury, often impacting an individual's emotional and psychological well-being for years to come. PTSD, a response to experiencing or witnessing a life-threatening event, can alter one's perception of safety, relationships, and even identity. It's essential to remember that PTSD isn't just a reaction to an event but a complex and ongoing process in which the mind attempts to make sense of overwhelming experiences. In fact, research has shown that trauma can literally change the brain's structure, affecting areas such as the hippocampus, which is involved in memory processing, and the amygdala, which plays a role in emotion regulation. This biological shift underscores the importance of understanding trauma not as a mere collection of symptoms, but as a reorganization of an individual's mental and emotional landscape.

One significant challenge in treating PTSD is that individuals may not always recognize their symptoms as a result of trauma. Symptoms can be subtle, such as a general sense of unease or difficulty concentrating, or they may present as more overt behaviors like hypervigilance or emotional numbing.

This variance can complicate the diagnostic process, often leading to misdiagnosis or delayed treatment. Furthermore, people with PTSD may not always be forthcoming about their experiences, either because of shame, fear, or simply not knowing how to articulate what they're going through. For those working in mental health care, it's critical to create a safe and nonjudgmental space where patients feel supported in sharing their stories. Only through trust and collaboration can effective healing begin.

Recent studies also highlight the wide-ranging impact of PTSD on physical health. Chronic stress from unresolved trauma can contribute to conditions like cardiovascular disease, autoimmune disorders, and chronic pain. These physical manifestations, often referred to as somatic symptoms, serve as a reminder of the body's connection to the mind and the profound effects of trauma on overall well-being. For health care providers, this means considering a holistic approach to treatment, addressing both the psychological and physical consequences of trauma.

Integrating therapies such as mindfulness, physical activity, and nutrition into treatment plans can significantly enhance the healing process, as they support the body's ability to recover from the physiological effects of stress.

Finally, it's important to recognize that recovery from PTSD is not linear. Healing is a multifaceted journey that involves setbacks and progress in equal measure. Some days may feel like a victory, while others may seem like a return to the beginning. However, research in trauma recovery shows that with the right interventions—whether through therapy, medication, or community support—resilience is not only possible but can thrive. Educating both professionals and the public about PTSD can help reduce stigma and foster a more compassionate and understanding environment for those affected. Ultimately, our collective knowledge and empathy are key in supporting individuals as they reclaim their lives, their relationships, and their mental well-being.

Overview of Symptoms

Post-Traumatic Stress Disorder (PTSD) manifests in myriad ways, reflecting a complex interplay of emotional, cognitive, and physiological disturbances. It's crucial to understand these symptoms not just as indicators of distress, but as profound signals of the impact of trauma on the human psyche. By identifying and understanding these symptoms, mental health professionals can better structure their therapeutic approaches, facilitating healing and empowerment for those affected.

One of the hallmark symptoms of PTSD is re-experiencing the traumatic event. This can occur in the form of vivid, intrusive memories, flashbacks, or distressing dreams. For individuals, these episodes can be profoundly disorienting, often accompanied by intense emotional and physiological reactions that can feel as vivid as the original trauma itself. The unpredictability and intensity of these re-experiences can severely disrupt a person's daily functioning and sense of safety.

Avoidance behaviors are another key symptom category, where individuals might go to great lengths to avoid reminders of the traumatic event. This can manifest as avoiding certain places, people, conversations, or even thoughts and feelings related to the trauma. While avoidance can offer temporary relief, it often exacerbates the condition, as it prevents individuals from processing the trauma in a healthy way. It's both a defense mechanism and a barrier to therapeutic progress, reinforcing the need for gentle yet deliberate therapeutic intervention.

Cognitive and mood disturbances are also prevalent among those with PTSD. This symptom category includes persistent negative beliefs about oneself, others, or the world, such as feelings of hopelessness, shame, or distrust. These core cognitive distortions can lead to feelings of detachment from society and a marked decrease in the ability to experience positive emotions. Such pervasive negative thinking patterns amplify the distress and complicate the therapeutic journey toward recovery.

The heightened state of arousal and reactivity is another facet of PTSD that contributes to the individual's distress and functional impairment. This might include symptoms like irritability, reckless or self-destructive behavior, exaggerated startle responses, problems with concentration, and difficulty sleeping. These hyperarousal symptoms keep individuals on high alert, often interfering with the ability to relax or concentrate on daily tasks, reflecting the body and mind's struggle to regain equilibrium after trauma.

To offer a comprehensive understanding of PTSD symptoms, it's also important to consider the cultural and individual contexts in which these symptoms develop. Symptom expression can vary significantly based on personal, cultural, and societal factors, requiring sensitive and nuanced approaches in both diagnosis and treatment. Mental health professionals need to be attuned to these variations to provide culturally competent care that respects individual differences.

Thus, a thorough grasp of PTSD symptoms is essential for mental health professionals not only to facilitate accurate diagnosis but also to inform the development of effective, individualized treatment plans. A nuanced understanding allows practitioners to better assist their clients in navigating the complexities of their experiences, promoting a sense of agency and empowerment in their healing journeys.Furthermore, it's vital for clinicians and educators to remain engaged with the latest research and evidence-based practices regarding PTSD symptoms. Advancements in neuroscientific and psychological understanding offer exciting possibilities for refining therapeutic techniques and improving outcomes for individuals with PTSD. Such knowledge empowers professionals to approach these symptoms with both empathy and expertise, ultimately guiding individuals toward greater resilience and recovery.

Addressing PTSD symptoms is not just about reducing distress but also fostering growth and healing. Acknowledging the human capacity for resilience and adaptation is essential. These insights on symptoms highlight not only the challenges faced by those affected but also the opportunities for healing and transformation available through dedicated, empathetic, and informed care.

Diagnosis Criteria

Understanding the diagnosis criteria for PTSD is foundational for mental health professionals as they navigate the complexities of treatment and support for their patients. Recognizing the symptoms is only the beginning. PTSD diagnosis requires a comprehensive assessment that adheres to established criteria, ensuring accuracy in identifying this challenging condition.

PTSD is characterized by a set of criteria outlined in the *Diagnostic and Statistical Manual of Mental Disorders* (DSM-5), which simplifies the understanding of this multifaceted disorder into clear, diagnostic components. The first criterion involves exposure to a traumatic event. This doesn't just mean experiencing the event but also witnessing it, learning about it happening to a close family member or friend, or being exposed to details of the trauma repeatedly. It's crucial for clinicians to recognize that the nature of exposure can vary widely between patients.

The second criterion focuses on intrusion symptoms. These are involuntary and recurrent memories, dreams, or flashbacks of the traumatic event. The emotional and physiological arousal accompanying these intrusions can significantly disrupt a patient's life. As professionals, acknowledging the impact these symptoms have on daily functioning is essential for empathizing with the patient's lived experience.

Next, there are persistent avoidance symptoms. This involves efforts to avoid thoughts, feelings, or external reminders of the trauma. These avoidance behaviors can become barriers to seeking or engaging in therapy, necessitating sensitive approaches by clinicians to guide patients towards safer, gradual exposure to these avoided elements.

Cognition and mood alterations form another essential diagnostic area. Patients may experience negative changes in their beliefs about themselves or others, emotional numbing, or an inability to remember critical aspects of the traumatic event. These are more than just mood disturbances—they can reshape a person's worldview. Health professionals must adeptly navigate these shifts to foster healing and trust.

The fourth criterion is marked by changes in arousal and reactivity. This includes hyper-vigilance, exaggerated startle responses, irritability, and difficulties with concentration or sleep. These symptoms can be both exhausting and alienating for the patient, often exacerbating feelings of isolation. Therapists must utilize strategies that help manage these heightened states and provide avenues for relief.

In addition to meeting these symptom clusters, the DSM-5 specifies that these disturbances must last more than a month and cause significant distress or impairment in social, occupational, or other important areas of functioning. Therefore, the duration and severity of symptoms are key factors in differentiating PTSD from other trauma-related disorders.

Moreover, the symptoms should not be attributable to the physiological effects of a substance or another medical condition. Ruling out these factors requires a thorough assessment process, underscoring the importance of comprehensive evaluation protocols in clinical settings.

While standardized diagnostic criteria provide a framework, they must be applied with clinical judgment. Professionals need to consider each person's unique context—life circumstances, cultural background, and personal history all contribute to how PTSD manifests and how the healing process can be most effectively initiated.

The variability in individual experiences of trauma underscores the importance of personalized diagnosis. It's not just about ticking boxes but understanding each patient's story and how they relate to their symptoms. This deeper understanding allows mental health practitioners to tailor interventions that align with the patient's personal and cultural needs.

The nuanced nature of PTSD diagnosis necessitates a well-rounded approach from clinicians. An accurate diagnosis sets the stage for effective intervention and creates a path for patients to reclaim their mental health. With careful attention to the diagnostic criteria, therapists can provide compassionate support, helping patients move from a place of suffering towards one of empowerment and recovery.

The impact of cultural factors on PTSD diagnosis cannot be overstated. For instance, certain cultures may emphasize communal support and may view trauma as something to be processed collectively, rather than individually. In contrast, more individualistic cultures might place a greater emphasis on personal resilience and self-reliance, potentially leading individuals to minimize their symptoms or avoid seeking help. By acknowledging and respecting these cultural nuances, mental health professionals can avoid misinterpretation of symptoms and ensure that the diagnosis reflects the individual's lived reality. Additionally, some cultures may have unique expressions or understanding of emotional distress, which could manifest in somatic symptoms, such as chronic pain or gastrointestinal issues, rather than the more commonly recognized psychological symptoms. Being aware of such differences can be key to providing appropriate care and avoiding the risk of overlooking or misdiagnosing PTSD.

Trauma-informed care is another crucial aspect that enhances the diagnostic process. Adopting a trauma-informed approach means recognizing the pervasive effects of trauma on both the patient and the clinician. Research has shown that trauma can impact memory, decision-making, and emotional regulation, all of which can influence how a person interacts with a clinician during assessment. By creating an environment that feels safe and non-threatening, clinicians can help reduce the risk of retraumatization and allow patients to feel more comfortable sharing their experiences. Additionally, trauma-informed care encourages clinicians to continuously reflect on their own biases and practices, fostering a more empathetic and effective approach to diagnosis. This perspective ensures that individuals with PTSD are not only diagnosed accurately but also treated with dignity and respect throughout their healing journey.

Impact on Daily Life

The impact of PTSD on daily life can be pervasive, influencing numerous aspects of an individual's personal and professional existence. It often acts as an invisible weight, affecting the mind and body in ways both subtle and overt. People dealing with PTSD encounter disruptions in their daily routines, relationships, and overall quality of life. This complex interplay of symptoms directly links to the difficulties they face, often making mundane tasks feel insurmountable.

Sleep disturbances are a common feature of PTSD, leading to chronic fatigue and a diminished capacity for concentration or patience. Insomnia or nightmares not only rob individuals of rest but also create a vicious cycle where anxiety about not sleeping exacerbates the problem. This often results in a general sense of irritability or frustration during the daytime, affecting work performance and social interactions. The lack of restful sleep can also contribute to heightened alertness and responsiveness to perceived threats, making typical environments feel overwhelming or unsafe.

Emotional numbness, another hallmark of PTSD, deeply affects social engagements. Individuals might withdraw from family gatherings, friendships, or work-related events, finding it hard to connect emotionally with others. This withdrawal isn't simply a matter of preference but a defensive mechanism to maintain some semblance of control over an unpredictable emotional landscape. The fear of being overwhelmed by emotions or triggering a traumatic memory can severely limit social involvement, leading to isolation and loneliness. Personal relationships often suffer as individuals with PTSD may appear detached or indifferent to those around them. Patience and understanding from loved ones become critical in maintaining these strained connections.

The cognitive impairments associated with PTSD, such as memory issues or difficulties in concentration, manifest in various life domains. This can be particularly debilitating in professional settings where sustained attention and effective communication are paramount. Mistakes in judgment or forgotten tasks can erode confidence, reducing job satisfaction or posing challenges in career advancement. The added stress of trying to maintain an adequate performance level can lead to anxiety and a decrease in overall mental health.

PTSD also impacts the individual's physical health, influencing both lifestyle choices and wellbeing. Those grappling with intrusive thoughts or hyperarousal may engage in unhealthy coping mechanisms such as substance use, poor eating habits, or sedentary behavior. Consequently, these behaviors may lead to chronic health issues such as obesity, cardiovascular disease, or diabetes, further complicating the individual's recovery and overall treatment plan. The interplay between mental and physical health necessitates a comprehensive therapeutic approach addressing both areas concurrently.

Financial stability may also be impacted as a result of PTSD. The difficulty in maintaining steady employment due to absenteeism, decreased productivity, or job loss can lead to financial strain. Worrying about financial issues can, in turn, exacerbate the symptoms of PTSD, creating a cycle of stress and instability. This financial stress can affect family dynamics, making it a critical area to address in therapy and support systems.

For individuals with PTSD, particularly parents, managing family responsibilities and child-rearing can pose specific challenges. The symptoms of PTSD may interfere with parenting roles and the ability to provide emotional support to children. This can have wider implications for family relationships and the emotional health of dependents. Ensuring that parents with PTSD have access to appropriate therapeutic resources can be beneficial in maintaining the family unit's health.

Given these myriad challenges, it is important for healthcare providers to recognize the profound and varied effects of PTSD on daily life. Effective management involves understanding and addressing these broad impacts —not just the symptoms of PTSD, but the ways in which these symptoms permeate and disrupt daily functioning. By doing so, interventions can be more tailored, creating more targeted and efficacious treatment plans that respect the uniqueness of each individual's experience.

The journey toward healing can be a long and challenging path, yet with the appropriate clinical support and personal resilience, individuals can reclaim their lives, finding the strength to confront and manage their PTSD. Healthcare professionals play a pivotal role in this transformative journey, offering guidance and fostering an empathetic environment for recovery.

In summary, PTSD is more than the sum of its symptoms. It is an all- encompassing force that can alter every facet of an individual's day-to-day life. Understanding its impact means recognizing the full extent of its reach, and acknowledging the courage it takes for survivors to strive towards healing and reclaiming their space. This understanding is crucial in providing the supportive, comprehensive care these individuals truly deserve.

The journey toward healing from PTSD requires a comprehensive approach that addresses both the psychological and practical aspects of an individual's life. Beyond addressing the core symptoms of trauma, effective management must consider how PTSD affects social relationships, employment, and day-to-day functioning. For example, individuals with PTSD may struggle with trust issues, leading to strained relationships with family, friends, and coworkers. These interpersonal challenges can exacerbate feelings of isolation and loneliness, making the healing process even more difficult. Furthermore, the symptoms of hypervigilance and avoidance can make navigating everyday situations, such as grocery shopping or attending social events, overwhelming. By recognizing these disruptions, healthcare providers can collaborate with patients to develop strategies that help reintegrate them into their daily routines in manageable ways. These targeted interventions may include social skills training, mindfulness techniques, or gradual exposure to feared situations, all of which can help restore a sense of control and autonomy in the face of overwhelming symptoms.

Moreover, research into trauma recovery has revealed that a strong support network, whether from family, friends, or peer groups, significantly influences outcomes in PTSD treatment. One fascinating study showed that people with PTSD who engaged in peer support groups reported lower levels of distress and improved coping mechanisms.

These findings highlight the importance of community and connection in the healing process. Mental health professionals can play a critical role in facilitating these connections, whether through group therapy, referrals to support networks, or by helping patients foster new social connections. Encouraging patients to rebuild their social networks and seek support from others who understand their experiences not only helps combat the feelings of isolation that often accompany PTSD but also strengthens the resilience needed for long-term recovery. Ultimately, by acknowledging the full breadth of PTSD's effects, healthcare providers can offer more holistic and empowering care, helping individuals to reclaim their lives and embrace their potential for healing.

CHAPTER 2

FOUNDATIONS OF COGNITIVE PROCESSING THERAPY (CPT)

Stepping into the world of Cognitive Processing Therapy (CPT), one begins by understanding its robust foundation, designed with precision to guide those entangled in the aftermath of trauma. It's not just a methodology, but a beacon of hope. Rooted in a historical context that sought to address gaps left by earlier therapeutic approaches, CPT stands on core principles that challenge distorted beliefs and fosters cognitive restructuring. The transformation it offers is layered, advocating for change through empirical evidence that reinforces its effectiveness. CPT empowers mental health professionals to tailor interventions that are compassionate yet firmly grounded in science, creating a pathway for individuals to reclaim their stories and rebuild their lives. In this chapter, we'll intertwine the clinical rigor with an empathetic approach, ensuring a comprehensive understanding of how CPT can fundamentally alter the trajectory of healing.

Cognitive Processing Therapy (CPT) emerged as an innovative response to the limitations of earlier trauma-focused therapies, particularly in its ability to address the cognitive distortions that often trap individuals in the cycle of PTSD. Traditional talk therapies often failed to address the specific thought patterns that contribute to the perpetuation of trauma-related distress, leaving patients vulnerable to the reactivation of painful memories and emotional triggers. CPT was developed to fill this gap, helping individuals to not only confront traumatic events but also to reframe the negative beliefs they developed as a result of those events. One of the key elements of CPT is its focus on identifying and challenging "stuck points"—negative beliefs about oneself, the world, or others that are rooted in trauma. Through this process, individuals can begin to understand how these beliefs shape their reactions and emotions, ultimately opening the door for healing and self-compassion.

At its core, CPT is structured to be both accessible and effective, providing a clear roadmap for patients to engage in their healing journey. Unlike some other therapies that require long-term commitment or extensive timeframes to see results, CPT is designed as a relatively brief intervention, often completed in about 12 sessions. This efficiency doesn't undermine its depth; rather, it highlights the therapy's ability to facilitate real and lasting change in a short period.

Research has shown that CPT leads to significant reductions in PTSD symptoms, with many individuals experiencing lasting improvements even months after completing therapy. The cognitive restructuring in CPT helps individuals move from a place of self-blame or guilt to one of understanding and self-acceptance, allowing them to regain control over their lives. Studies indicate that these changes in thought patterns are often linked to improved emotional regulation, better interpersonal relationships, and greater overall functioning.

CPT's adaptability is another factor that has contributed to its widespread success. While it was originally developed for individuals with PTSD related to sexual assault and military combat, it has since been shown to be effective across a broad range of trauma types, including natural disasters, childhood abuse, and accidents. This versatility makes CPT an invaluable tool for clinicians who are working with diverse populations. Not only can CPT be tailored to address the specific trauma experienced by an individual, but it can also be adapted for different delivery formats, including individual therapy, group therapy, and even online therapy platforms. For example, recent studies have demonstrated the effectiveness of online CPT programs for people who may have limited access to in-person therapy due to geographical constraints or social stigma. This expanding reach highlights the importance of making trauma-informed care accessible to a wider audience.

Additionally, one of the most powerful aspects of CPT is the therapeutic alliance it fosters between the clinician and the patient. While the therapy's focus on cognitive restructuring is central, the relationship between therapist and patient plays a crucial role in the success of the treatment. A compassionate and empathetic therapist helps create a safe space where patients feel supported as they confront their trauma.

The shared experience of identifying and challenging deeply held beliefs about the self and the world builds trust and encourages emotional vulnerability. This, in turn, accelerates the healing process, as patients feel validated and empowered in their journey toward recovery. Research consistently supports the idea that the quality of the therapeutic relationship in trauma treatment is one of the strongest predictors of positive outcomes, reinforcing the importance of an approach that balances both clinical expertise and empathetic care.

Historical Background

The origins of Cognitive Processing Therapy (CPT) as a therapeutic approach for post-traumatic stress disorder (PTSD) are deeply rooted in the broader historical context of cognitive-behavioral therapy (CBT) and the evolving understanding of trauma and its psychological impacts. To appreciate the transformative power of CPT, it's essential to trace its development through decades of research and theoretical advancements.

In the mid-20th century, the cognitive revolution began to shift the landscape of psychology. This period marked a departure from behaviorism, emphasizing the role of internal mental processes. Albert Ellis and Aaron Beck, significant figures during this time, developed foundational cognitive theories and therapies. Ellis's Rational Emotive Behavior Therapy (REBT) and Beck's Cognitive Therapy (CT) highlighted how cognition influences emotions and behavior. These theories laid the groundwork for the later development of therapies focusing on modifying maladaptive thought patterns, setting the stage for CPT.

Understanding trauma and its pervasive effects found increased focus during and after the Vietnam War. The psychological toll on veterans propelled trauma into the public and academic discourse. This period saw the conceptualization and eventual acceptance of PTSD as a clinical diagnosis in the third edition of the Diagnostic and Statistical Manual of Mental Disorders (DSM-III) in 1980. This recognition paved the way for developing specialized therapies tailored to the unique challenges faced by trauma survivors.

By the 1980s, there was a growing recognition of the need for targeted interventions for trauma. Patricia Resick, a pioneering figure in trauma therapy, began to develop CPT as a structured approach to address PTSD symptoms. Her work integrated cognitive-behavioral principles with insights specific to trauma's multifaceted nature, focusing on the distorted beliefs and interpretations that often follow traumatic experiences. CPT emphasized the idea that changing how one perceives and processes trauma can significantly alleviate PTSD symptoms.

CPT's initial development was also influenced by the evolving understanding of how trauma affects memory and cognition. Research had started to uncover how trauma can disrupt cognitive processes, leading to intrusive thoughts, avoidance behaviors, and emotional numbing. By addressing these disruptions, CPT aimed to help individuals reconstruct their trauma narratives in a way that promotes healing and recovery.

The effectiveness of CPT gained empirical support through rigorous clinical trials, primarily focusing on populations with significant exposure to trauma, such as military veterans and survivors of sexual assault. These studies not only validated CPT as an evidence-based practice but also highlighted its adaptability across various demographic groups and trauma types. This adaptability helped CPT gain widespread recognition and adoption in both clinical settings and academic circles.

The 1990s and early 2000s saw a proliferation of research validating CPT's mechanisms. Studies demonstrated how CPT effectively targets cognitive disruptions and maladaptive beliefs, facilitating healthier processing of traumatic memories. This period was marked by refinements in protocol and a deeper understanding of cognitive restructuring techniques, making CPT a cornerstone in trauma therapy.

The historical progression of CPT is also marked by its inclusion in treatment guidelines by prominent organizations such as the Department of Veterans Affairs and the Department of Defense. These endorsements underscored CPT's efficacy and importance in addressing trauma-related disorders, reflecting a broader acceptance within the therapeutic community.

Today, the historical legacy of CPT is evident in its ongoing evolution and implementation in diverse settings. The therapy continues to adapt, incorporating new research findings and technological advancements to enhance its effectiveness. It stands as a testament to the dynamic interplay between cognitive theory, empirical research, and the compassionate desire to help individuals reclaim their lives from the grips of trauma.

The validation of Cognitive Processing Therapy (CPT) during the 1990s and early 2000s not only demonstrated its effectiveness but also spurred a broader shift in trauma care. Researchers began to refine their understanding of how PTSD manifests in the brain, particularly in areas such as memory processing and emotional regulation. Advances in neuroimaging allowed for the observation of how trauma affects brain structures like the hippocampus and amygdala, providing compelling evidence of the physiological changes that occur in response to trauma. CPT's ability to address these cognitive disruptions was further underscored by studies showing changes in brain activity and connectivity in patients who underwent the therapy. These findings solidified CPT as not just a psychological intervention, but as a treatment that aligned with emerging neurobiological understandings of trauma and recovery. This evidence-based approach also paved the way for CPT's adoption across various healthcare systems, contributing to its widespread use in military, civilian, and clinical settings alike.

As CPT's reputation grew, it became a key component in many national and international treatment protocols. The Department of Veterans Affairs and the Department of Defense played pivotal roles in championing CPT as a primary treatment for PTSD, particularly for veterans returning from conflict zones like Iraq and Afghanistan. Their endorsement was based on extensive research demonstrating CPT's ability to reduce PTSD symptoms and improve overall mental health, especially in populations dealing with combat-related trauma. Furthermore, the inclusion of CPT in these treatment guidelines was a crucial moment in mental health care, signaling a move toward evidence-based practices that prioritize both the science of healing and the lived experience of those affected by trauma. This commitment to research-informed care has continued to shape the landscape of trauma therapy, ensuring that interventions like CPT remain at the forefront of trauma recovery and continue to evolve alongside emerging therapeutic and technological advancements.

Core Principles of CPT

Cognitive Processing Therapy (CPT) stands as a beacon for addressing and treating Post-Traumatic Stress Disorder (PTSD). At its core, it's a structured, evidence-based therapeutic approach grounded in cognitive- behavioral techniques. The principles of CPT focus on transforming the way individuals perceive and process traumatic events, offering a pathway to healing and resilience. Let's dive into these core principles with an understanding of their profound impact on mental health recovery.

The primary principle of CPT is the recognition of the relationship between thoughts, emotions, and behaviors following trauma. Traumatic events can often rewrite our cognitive landscape, trapping us in cycles of distressing thoughts and emotions. CPT provides tools to examine these thoughts critically and understand how they influence our emotional and behavioral responses. By doing so, individuals can identify and challenge maladaptive beliefs, opening doors to new perspectives and healthier emotional states.

Acknowledging and dissecting "stuck points" is another cornerstone of CPT. These are thoughts related to the trauma that persistently intrude and disrupt daily life. For example, a survivor might ruminate on thoughts like "It was my fault" or "I'm not safe anywhere." In therapy, these stuck points are not just identified but rigorously examined in light of objective evidence. The therapist guides the individual in questioning the validity of these thoughts, encouraging a shift toward more balanced, adaptive beliefs.

Moreover, CPT emphasizes the therapeutic power of writing and verbal processing. Clients are often encouraged to write detailed accounts of their traumatic experiences. This process isn't merely recounting events; it's an opportunity to engage deeply with the memories, examining the emotions and thoughts that arise. Through this narrative reconstruction, clients can confront and reframe their traumatic narratives, which can significantly reduce the power these memories hold over them.

Another core principle involves understanding how trauma impacts one's belief systems about safety, trust, power, esteem, and intimacy. Traumatic experiences can dramatically alter these fundamental beliefs, often leading to generalized and distorted views about oneself and the world. CPT systematically explores these shifts, helping clients to rebuild a belief system that more accurately reflects reality and promotes psychological well-being.

CPT also highlights the importance of collaboration and active participation. Unlike more passive therapeutic approaches, CPT requires the client to be actively engaged in their healing process. This collaborative nature empowers the individual, fostering a sense of agency and control over their recovery journey. The therapist acts as a facilitator and guide, providing the structure and support necessary for the client to explore their thoughts and emotions thoroughly.

Furthermore, CPT acknowledges the cultural, social, and individual nuances of each client, tailoring interventions to meet unique needs. This principle underscores the adaptability of CPT, ensuring that therapeutic interventions are not only effective but also culturally sensitive. The approach respects diverse perspectives and experiences, aligning treatment with the client's personal and cultural context.

In essence, the core principles of CPT are rooted in empowerment and transformation. By systematically addressing the cognitive processes disrupted by trauma, CPT empowers individuals to reclaim their mental space and time. It encourages them to move beyond the constraints of their past experiences, fostering resilience and a renewed sense of hope.

Incorporating these core principles, CPT offers a pathway not only to alleviate the symptoms of PTSD but also to nurture a deeper understanding of the self and the world. For healthcare providers, researchers, and mental health professionals, embracing these principles means fostering environments where clients feel safe, understood, and supported as they navigate their paths to recovery. Through empathic guidance and structured interventions, CPT stands as a powerful testament to the transformative possibilities of therapy.

Evidence-Based Research

Understanding the foundations of Cognitive Processing Therapy (CPT) requires delving into the empirical evidence that supports its efficacy. This section lays the groundwork for practitioners and researchers to appreciate the robust scientific backing of CPT, a therapy extensively employed for individuals grappling with Post-Traumatic Stress Disorder (PTSD). Across various settings and populations, evidence-based research offers a window into why CPT remains a cornerstone for trauma-focused therapies.

The first promising data emerged from the initial clinical trials conducted in the late 1980s and early 1990s. These studies sought to examine the effectiveness of CPT among sexual assault survivors who exhibited PTSD symptoms. The results were compelling, showing marked reductions in PTSD symptoms at a level greater than those experienced through supportive therapies alone. Early trials focused on finding tangible outcomes such as reduced symptoms and increased daily functioning, which laid the framework for larger research endeavors.

As the body of research grew, so did the diverse applications of CPT. It wasn't long before researchers extended its use to a variety of trauma types and settings. Studies involving combat veterans, for instance, revealed CPT's profound impact on this unique demographic. Not only did participants report lower PTSD symptoms post-treatment, but they also experienced improvements in depression, anger, and guilt. These multidimensional benefits highlighted CPT's holistic approach to trauma recovery.

Meta-analyses play a crucial role in supporting the efficacy of CPT. By pooling data from numerous studies, these analyses demonstrate significantly higher effect sizes for CPT compared to other therapeutic interventions. The aggregated data provides compelling evidence of CPT's broad-spectrum efficacy, confirming its status as a gold-standard treatment for PTSD. Such meta-analyses underscore the consistent and robust outcomes that CPT offers across different populations and varying types of trauma.

In recent years, the focus of research has shifted towards understanding the mechanisms through which CPT facilitates change. Cognitive restructuring, a core component of CPT, activates key neural pathways involved in emotion regulation and cognitive control. Neuroimaging studies shed light on how CPT modifies brain activity patterns, suggesting that changes at the cognitive level translate into neurological adjustments. These findings invigorate the argument for CPT, aligning cognitive theory with empirical observations of brain plasticity.

A critical aspect of CPT's evidence base revolves around its adaptability and effectiveness within diverse populations. Research endeavors focusing on cultural competence and sensitivity have shown that CPT can be tailored to accommodate cultural and individual differences without losing its therapeutic potency. Studies involving minority groups and immigrant populations have reported success, proving CPT's adaptability to various cultural contexts and underscoring the importance of culturally informed practice.

Furthermore, randomized controlled trials comparing CPT with other therapeutic modalities, such as prolonged exposure therapy and eye movement desensitization and reprocessing (EMDR), continue to affirm CPT's effectiveness. While each therapy has its strengths, CPT stands out for its structured approach, emphasizing the processing and restructuring of cognitive distortions. Comparative studies illustrate not just the efficacy of CPT, but its facilitating role in helping patients confront and reframe their trauma narratives effectively.

Research into long-term outcomes provides additional insights into CPT's sustainability as a treatment option. Studies following participants months and even years after treatment conclude that the improvements made during CPT are often maintained. These enduring treatment outcomes reinforce CPT as an integral component of long-term PTSD management strategies and highlight its comprehensive benefits beyond the immediacy of symptom relief.

Innovative research methodologies, such as hybrid effectiveness- implementation trials, are paving the way for studying CPT in real-world settings. Such studies bridge the gap between controlled research environments and clinical practice, providing evidence that supports the integration of CPT into routine mental health care frameworks globally. This pragmatic research approach continues to validate CPT in diverse clinical settings, ensuring its relevance and applicability to future generations of therapists and patients.

Despite the plethora of positive findings, ongoing research is pivotal to address unanswered questions and improve CPT further. Emerging areas of interest include tailoring CPT for individuals with complex PTSD, adapting CPT for teletherapy frameworks as digital health gains traction, and optimizing treatment for co-occurring PTSD and substance use disorders. By continuing to expand our understanding of CPT through rigorous scientific inquiry, the field of trauma therapy can innovate and fine-tune approaches to meet the evolving needs of clients.

In conclusion, the evidence base of Cognitive Processing Therapy is both vast and compelling, establishing it as an empirically supported treatment for PTSD that mental health professionals rely on. Its capacity to facilitate meaningful, sustained recovery from trauma makes it indispensable in the therapeutic toolbox. For healthcare providers, clinical supervisors, educators, and researchers, embracing the evidence that underscores CPT is essential for advancing trauma-informed care and inspiring hope in the countless individuals who seek healing from the impacts of trauma.

CHAPTER 3

PREPARING FOR THERAPY

Preparing for therapy involves a thoughtful approach that is essential for creating a healing journey that is as impactful as it is effective. At the outset, initial assessments are crucial in understanding the unique stories and symptoms that each individual brings to the therapeutic setting. These assessments help tailor the therapeutic experience, ensuring that care is attuned to specific needs. Creating a safe environment goes beyond physical space; it involves cultivating an atmosphere where trust and openness can flourish, allowing individuals to engage deeply with the process. Setting therapy goals is another integral component, providing a roadmap that guides both the therapist and the individual through the emotional terrain they will traverse together. These objectives not only offer direction but also imbue the therapeutic process with purpose, inspiring individuals to reclaim their strength and resilience. Together, these foundational steps lay the groundwork for a therapeutic relationship that is both transformative and enduring.

The significance of the initial assessment cannot be overstated, as it provides the foundation for a personalized and effective therapeutic journey. In this phase, mental health professionals gather not only the clinical information necessary for diagnosis but also the nuanced details that paint a fuller picture of the person in front of them. Questions about past experiences, cultural background, and current life circumstances are integral to understanding how trauma has shaped the individual's worldview and coping strategies. This holistic approach ensures that the treatment plan is not one-size-fits-all, but instead is uniquely crafted to address the particularities of each person's trauma and healing process. Research supports the idea that individualized care significantly enhances treatment outcomes, as it fosters a deeper sense of connection and relevance for the patient, making them feel understood and respected in their healing journey.

Creating a safe environment is an essential step in preparing for therapy, and its importance extends far beyond the therapeutic setting itself.

The atmosphere of safety, both physical and emotional, fosters a sense of security that allows individuals to engage in vulnerable, often difficult, emotional work. Studies have shown that trust is a crucial predictor of therapeutic success, as patients are more likely to share deeply personal experiences when they feel protected from judgment and re-traumatization. Therapists can cultivate this sense of safety through active listening, empathy, and maintaining consistent boundaries that respect the patient's autonomy. This space for openness creates the conditions for meaningful change, as individuals are able to explore their trauma without fear, supported by the presence of a compassionate and skilled guide. Furthermore, setting clear therapy goals at the outset provides not only a sense of structure and purpose but also allows individuals to see progress as they move toward healing, reinforcing the belief that transformation is not only possible but achievable.

Initial Assessments

As professionals begin the therapeutic journey, the importance of initial assessments cannot be overstated. This crucial step sets the stage for the therapy process, providing both therapist and client with a comprehensive understanding of the issues at hand.

Through assessments, we begin to unravel the intricacies of each individual's experiences, paving the way for tailored therapeutic interventions.

Initial assessments serve as the compass guiding the therapeutic path. They are not merely checklists but dynamic, evolving conversations that bring to light the client's past and present. The assessment process should be approached with sensitivity and care, recognizing the courage it takes for clients to disclose their personal and often painful histories. In this phase, therapists are tasked with creating a space where clients feel seen, heard, and validated, which is instrumental in fostering a sense of safety and trust.

One of the primary goals during the initial assessments is to gather a thorough history. This involves exploring the client's background, including family dynamics, social relationships, and any significant life events that may have contributed to their current state. It is essential to understand the context of their trauma, as it allows therapists to better empathize with the client's experiences and adapt their approach accordingly. Gathering this information helps in formulating a working hypothesis about how the trauma has impacted the client's cognitive and emotional processes.

Despite its significance, the assessment phase should be balanced with patience and attentiveness to the client's readiness to share. Rushing this process could hinder the development of the therapeutic alliance. Instead, assessments should be an ongoing dialogue that evolves over time. This flexibility allows the therapist to respect the client's pace and accommodate any new concerns or insights that may arise throughout therapy.

Furthermore, recognizing the diversity of trauma experiences is crucial. An initial assessment is the perfect opportunity to address potential cultural, social, or individual differences that might affect how trauma manifests in different individuals. Tailoring the assessment process to these nuances can enhance the relevancy and effectiveness of the therapy that follows. Acknowledging these unique factors helps in understanding how trauma interacts with one's identity and personal narrative, which is fundamental in delivering culturally competent care.

Beyond gathering history, initial assessments should also focus on evaluating the client's current functioning. This includes an exploration of the symptoms they are experiencing, such as anxiety, depression, or hyper-vigilance, and how these symptoms disrupt their daily lives. Identifying the severity and frequency of these symptoms can help in setting realistic goals and tracking progress throughout the therapy. Quantitative measures, like standardized assessment tools, can be beneficial in capturing these details, providing a baseline that can be used to evaluate therapeutic outcomes.

In addition to establishing a clinical profile, initial assessments allow therapists to identify any immediate safety concerns. This includes assessing risks such as self-harm, suicidal ideation, or any other behaviors that might endanger the client or others. A comprehensive safety assessment is vital, as it ensures that clients receive the necessary interventions to manage these risks effectively.

Equally important is the assessment of the client's existing coping mechanisms and support systems. Understanding what resources and strategies clients are already utilizing can inform the therapy process, highlighting strengths and areas of resilience that can be built upon. It can also uncover maladaptive coping strategies that may need to be addressed to foster more effective behavioral patterns.

Assessments also offer an opportunity to begin exploring the client's goals and expectations for therapy. Engaging clients in this way promotes collaboration and empowers them to take an active role in their healing process. This marks the beginning of goal-setting, allowing for a mutual understanding of what therapeutic success looks like from the client's perspective. Aligning expectations from the outset can significantly impact the client's engagement and the overall efficacy of the treatment.

Above all, initial assessments should cultivate a space of empathy and compassion. They are the therapist's first chance to demonstrate an unconditional positive regard, setting a precedent for the therapeutic relationship. This foundation of trust allows clients to gradually open up, facilitating deeper exploration and eventual transformation. The therapist's role here is to listen intently, validate the client's experiences, and collaboratively embark on the journey towards healing.

Ultimately, the initial assessment phase is a significant investment in the therapeutic process. It not only establishes the framework for individualized therapy but also reinforces the therapeutic alliance. As such, healthcare providers, researchers, and graduate students should view this stage as a cornerstone of effective treatment, one that requires thoughtful consideration and intentional action.

By prioritizing comprehensive and empathetic initial assessments, mental health professionals can better serve their clients, empowering them to reclaim control of their lives and mental well-being. This essential step sets the tone for the entire therapeutic journey, ensuring that each path is as unique and multifaceted as the individuals who walk it.

Creating a Safe Environment

Creating a safe environment is fundamental in preparing for therapy, particularly for individuals grappling with trauma-related disorders. It's essential to realize that the physical and emotional surroundings in which therapy takes place can significantly influence the therapeutic outcomes. Clients need a space that radiates safety and trust, fostering an atmosphere where they're free to express and process intense emotions without fear of judgment or consequence.

Psychological safety is as important as the physical environment. The therapy room should be a haven from potential triggers. This can start with simple gestures, like ensuring comfortable seating and arranging the space to feel open but not overwhelming. Lighting and noise levels play a role in creating an inviting atmosphere, avoiding harsh fluorescent lights or loud, distracting sounds. What's paramount is the effort invested in making every client feel valued and heard right from their first session.

Establishing a safe therapeutic environment also requires keen attention to personal interactions. A therapist's demeanor can establish the trust bridge between them and their client. Simple practices such as active listening and validating a client's emotions can reinforce a sense of security. It's crucial for therapists to be genuine and consistent in their interactions, as clients can often detect when authenticity is lacking.

Safety in therapy is not solely reserved for the physical space or initial interactions; it also involves structuring the therapeutic sessions to foster predictability and control. Clients should be informed about what to expect from therapy, including potential challenges they might face during the process. Outlining this process helps manage expectations and reduces anxiety, allowing clients to engage more fully with the therapeutic work.

Confidentiality is another cornerstone of creating a safe environment. Clients must understand the extent and limitations of confidentiality in therapy. Assuring them that their disclosures are protected can facilitate more honest and meaningful dialogues. This assurance can be reinforced by frequent reminders about confidentiality, particularly when challenging subjects are broached.

Empathy should guide every therapeutic interaction. Engaging clients with empathy involves trying to understand their experiences and emotions without imposing one's own interpretations or judgments. It means accepting their stories and validating their feelings, fostering a safe emotional climate conducive to healing. Empathy encourages exploration and breakthrough as clients feel understood and accepted.

For many clients, especially those with post-traumatic stress disorder, safety is intricately tied with control. Empowering clients by actively involving them in the therapeutic process can diminish feelings of vulnerability. Therapists can facilitate this by collaboratively setting therapy goals and frequently soliciting feedback, allowing clients to steer the therapeutic journey.

These foundational aspects of creating a safe environment often bypass the conscious awareness of both the therapist and the client. Yet, they underpin the therapeutic relationship and can influence whether a client feels truly supported. On a broader scale, the principles of creating safety should permeate the entire therapeutic practice, offering a model that recognizes the complexity and uniqueness of each client's journey.

It can be helpful to involve clients in the conversation about what makes them feel safe. Each individual's experience with trauma is different, necessitating unique approaches to establishing safety. Discussing these topics openly can also empower clients, giving them a voice in their therapeutic process. It's a crucial part of developing a therapeutic alliance that is both resilient and responsive.

Moreover, therapists need to remain vigilant about the dynamics of the therapeutic environment and ready to adapt to any changes that could impinge on a client's sense of safety. Consistent reflection and supervision can support therapists in maintaining this vigilance. By routinely examining both personal and environmental influences on therapy, therapists can continue to refine the therapeutic setting to maximize efficacy.

Safety extends beyond the client-therapist interactions and includes considerations for clients' ongoing journeys. Checking in on their progress and providing them with resources to manage potential distress outside of sessions reinforces the safety net established within therapy. Crisis planning, for example, ensures clients have practical tools and strategies available if they encounter severe distress.

Ultimately, the creation of a safe environment in therapy is not a static goal but an ongoing process. It is a dynamic interplay between the therapist's presence, the therapeutic setting, and the client's evolving needs. The pursuit of safety is a testament to the therapist's commitment to fostering a space where profound healing can occur.

Setting Therapy Goals

Stepping into the realm of therapy can be daunting for both the patient and the therapist. To navigate this journey effectively, setting clear and meaningful therapy goals is crucial. Goals provide direction and purpose, creating a roadmap that guides each session and anchors the therapeutic process. They act as milestones, marking progress and highlighting areas where focus is needed. The collaborative effort in setting these goals can significantly enhance the therapeutic alliance and empower patients in their healing journey.

When setting therapy goals, it's vital to begin with a comprehensive understanding of the patient's personal experiences and the impact of trauma on their life. This understanding forms the foundation for realistic and personalized goals that reflect the patient's values and aspirations. Goals should be specific, measurable, achievable, relevant, and time- bound (SMART), helping patients focus on manageable steps that lead to larger therapeutic outcomes. Rather than overwhelming the patient with the enormity of recovery, SMART goals break down the process into tangible actions.

A patient-centered approach to goal-setting allows individuals to have a say in their healing process, fostering a sense of ownership and autonomy. This empowerment is a therapeutic tool in itself, helping individuals overcome feelings of helplessness and instilling hope. The therapist plays a crucial role in facilitating this process, providing guidance and expertise while respecting the patient's knowledge of their own needs and limitations.

It is also important to acknowledge that therapy goals may evolve over time. As patients gain insight and make progress, their priorities and needs might shift. Flexibility is key. Therapists should regularly revisit and adjust goals, ensuring they remain aligned with the patient's evolving understanding of their trauma and recovery. This dynamic process not only enhances the therapeutic experience but also encourages patients to engage more actively, knowing that their goals and ambitions are dynamic, just like their healing journey.

The therapist's role in this journey is multi-faceted. They must ensure a balance between challenging the patient to foster growth and providing the necessary support to handle setbacks. This equilibrium is often achieved through careful pacing, empathetic communication, and active listening. By cultivating an environment of trust and respect, therapists can help patients confront difficult emotions and beliefs that are pivotal to their recovery.

Moreover, setting therapy goals is an opportunity to identify and address barriers that may impede progress. These can be internal, such as self- doubt or fear of change, or external, such as lack of resources or support systems. By acknowledging these hurdles early in the therapeutic process, therapists and patients can collaboratively develop strategies to overcome them, ensuring a smoother path toward goal attainment.

The impact of setting therapy goals extends beyond the confines of the therapy session. It equips patients with skills that they can apply in various aspects of their lives, fostering a sense of agency that can be transformative. The ability to set and achieve goals is a critical component of personal development and self-efficacy, empowering individuals to navigate life's challenges with resilience and confidence.

In conclusion, setting therapy goals is a fundamental component of preparing for therapy. It requires a collaborative effort that blends the therapist's professional insights with the patient's lived experience. Together, therapist and patient can create a roadmap that not only guides the therapeutic process but also empowers the patient to reclaim their time and mental space, laying the groundwork for a fulfilling and healed life.

CHAPTER 4

COGNITIVE THEORY AND TRAUMA

In bridging the gap between trauma experiences and cognitive theory, it's crucial to recognize how deeply intertwined our belief systems and thought patterns are with the aftermath of trauma. Trauma doesn't just leave a mark on one's memory; it reshapes the lens through which they view the world. Our cognitive models play a pivotal role in this transformation, as they dictate how we process and interpret traumatic events.

Often, these thought patterns become distorted, leading to persistent and maladaptive beliefs that challenge recovery. By understanding and addressing these cognitive processes, mental health professionals are not only helping individuals navigate their trauma but also empowering them to reclaim control over their mental space. This journey involves unraveling these deeply rooted beliefs and gently guiding patients towards healthier, more adaptive perspectives. As we delve into these cognitive intricacies, remember that this is about equipping patients, supporting their resilience, and ultimately fostering a sense of hope and agency in their healing journey.

Cognitive Models in PTSD

In the intricate landscape of trauma and its psychological impacts, cognitive models serve as vital instruments, illuminating how post- traumatic stress disorder (PTSD) unfurls within the human mind.

These cognitive frameworks are not merely theoretical constructs; they guide practitioners in unraveling the complexities of PTSD, offering insight into why some individuals develop PTSD while others, exposed to similar traumas, do not. For health care providers, researchers, and mental health professionals, understanding these models is a crucial step in empowering patients to navigate their mental landscapes with clarity and resilience.

Cognitive models in PTSD primarily focus on the role of thought patterns and their interplay with emotional and behavioral responses following trauma. At the core, these models posit that it is not solely the trauma itself that dictates the emergence of PTSD symptoms, but rather the individual's interpretation and processing of that trauma. This distinction opens a realm of possibilities for intervention, where the modification of thought patterns can alter the trajectory of PTSD.

Central to these models is the concept of **cognitive processing theory**, which suggests that PTSD arises from disruptions in information processing. Trauma can shatter the previously held beliefs about safety, trust, control, esteem, and intimacy. When these foundational beliefs are challenged, a person may struggle to reconcile their new reality, resulting in maladaptive thoughts and behaviors. By acknowledging this disruption, cognitive models provide a roadmap for restructuring these thoughts and beliefs, aiming to restore a coherent sense of self and the world.

The work of therapists in this context becomes transformational. They serve as guides, helping patients sift through the rubble of their post- trauma world. Professionals leverage cognitive models to identify patterns of re-experiencing, avoidance, and hyperarousal, which are hallmark symptoms of PTSD. Through this lens, therapy becomes an empowering process aimed at fostering resilience, rather than a simple remediation of symptoms.

One influential cognitive model is *Emotional Processing Theory*, proposed by Edna Foa and Michael Kozak. This model delves into the idea that fear structures formed in response to trauma include information about the feared stimuli, responses to this fear, and the meaning of such stimuli and responses. When these structures are activated, typical outcomes include intrusive re-experiencing of memories and hyper- alertness to reminders of trauma. Emotional processing involves engaging with these fear structures, inviting patients to confront their discomfort in a controlled, therapeutic environment. This approach not only seeks to diminish PTSD symptoms but aims to reconcile emotional responses with reality-based interpretations of the trauma.

Another valuable framework is the *Dual Representation Theory* (DRT) introduced by Chris Brewin. DRT posits that there are two types of memory representations involved in PTSD: verbally accessible memories (VAMs) and situationally accessible memories (SAMs). VAMs are easily retrievable and reflect processing during trauma. SAMs, however, are involuntary and get triggered by environmental cues, often without the individual's conscious awareness. By understanding these two forms of memory, therapists can target interventions to better integrate these representations, allowing both overt and covert trauma memories to be processed in a balanced manner.

Beyond memory and emotional processing, cognitive models emphasize the role of **belief systems**. Traumatic experiences often lead individuals to reconstruct their beliefs in fundamental ways, sometimes adopting negative worldviews. These distorted beliefs, in turn, exacerbate PTSD symptoms. For instance, someone might develop an over-generalized belief that the world is perpetually dangerous or that they themselves are incapable of self-protection. Addressing and modifying these beliefs through cognitive restructuring can dramatically shift a patient's experience of anxiety and stress.

The practical implementation of cognitive models in therapy involves several techniques. One prominent method is *cognitive behavioral therapy* (CBT), which employs strategies such as cognitive restructuring and exposure therapy. CBT works by challenging distorted cognitions,

fostering adaptive thought patterns, and gradually exposing individuals to trauma-related stimuli in a controlled, therapeutic manner. The goal is not only symptom alleviation but the nurturing of psychological strength that can withstand future adversities.

Incorporating cognitive models also requires practitioners to possess acute empathy and adaptive communication skills. The therapist's role transcends from being a technique provider to a partner in the therapeutic journey, one who listens deeply and adapts interventions to the unique narratives and backgrounds of each patient. This humanistic approach underscores the inspirational potential of cognitive therapy: through understanding and reworking maladaptive thoughts, individuals reclaim agency over their mental lives.

Furthermore, cognitive models in PTSD are continually evolving. Research into the neurobiological underpinnings of trauma and cognition promises to refine these models, bringing forth even more precise and personalized therapeutic approaches. This progression underscores a hopeful message: with each scientific advancement, professionals are better equipped to guide individuals away from the shadows of trauma and towards a place of healing and wholeness.

For those engaged in the work of healing trauma, the cognitive models provide not only strategies but a profound sense of purpose. By applying these theories with empathy and expertise, they offer those affected by PTSD the possibility of transformation. The path to recovery is not easy, yet with each step informed by cognitive understanding, individuals can rebuild their lives, perhaps stronger than ever before. This synergy of science and compassion is where the journey towards reclaiming time and mental space truly begins.

Belief Systems and Trauma

Understanding belief systems and their relationship with trauma is a pivotal part of cognitive theory, particularly in the context of post- traumatic stress disorder (PTSD). Traumatic events can upheave an individual's foundational beliefs, often leading to a distorted worldview. This section aims to explore how these belief systems are shaped, challenged, and transformed in the aftermath of trauma, providing mental health professionals with insights to facilitate healing and recovery.

Beliefs are like the guiding stars of our perception—the lenses through which we see ourselves and the world. These beliefs form early in life and are molded by personal experiences, cultural influences, and social environments. They are usually stable and consistent, offering a sense of certainty and predictability. However, trauma can shatter these belief structures, leading to feelings of chaos and confusion. Consider a person who believes the world is a fundamentally safe place. A traumatic event can dismantle this notion, resulting in a profound sense of vulnerability and fear.

Cognitive theory posits that trauma can fundamentally alter core beliefs, such as those related to safety, trust, power, esteem, and intimacy. These changes often manifest as maladaptive thoughts, contributing to symptoms of PTSD. The intrusion of such cognitive distortions can perpetuate the cycle of trauma, affecting daily functioning and overall well-being. For example, survivors may begin to see themselves as inadequate or blame themselves for the trauma, believing they are unworthy of help or love. As healthcare providers, recognizing these shifts in belief is crucial to addressing the root cause of trauma-related distress.

Belief systems don't only exist in the abstract; they have tangible impacts on emotions and behaviors. For instance, if a person believes they are helpless, this belief can lead to avoidance behaviors typical in PTSD, where individuals shy away from situations that might challenge their entrenched views. Similarly, altered beliefs about trust can damage relationships, causing isolation and increasing the burden of psychological distress. The art of therapy, then, involves gently challenging these beliefs and guiding individuals to reconstruct their cognitive frameworks.

The therapeutic process should be empathetic and compassionate, focusing on creating a safe space for patients to explore and express their beliefs. Therapists might use techniques like Socratic questioning to help individuals examine their belief systems critically. This reflective method encourages patients to question the evidence supporting their beliefs, fostering cognitive flexibility and insight. Such interventions are not just about correcting faulty cognitions but also about empowering individuals to reclaim their sense of agency and control.

Trauma-informed care acknowledges that a changed belief system is not just a symptom to be fixed but a crucial part of the individual's trauma narrative. Therapists must be aware of their own biases and cultural backgrounds, which can shape their perception of patients' belief systems. Understanding and respecting the cultural contexts and individual differences of patients can significantly enhance the therapeutic alliance and the effectiveness of cognitive interventions.

Moreover, the collaborative nature of therapy enables patients to play an active role in their recovery journey. By acknowledging and validating their experiences and emotions, therapists can help patients reframe their narratives in a way that aligns with healthier and more adaptive beliefs. This empowerment process encourages patients to view their trauma as part of their life story but not define who they are. It allows them to rediscover their strengths and build resilience in the face of future adversities.

It's crucial for therapists to remember that changing belief systems is not an overnight endeavor. The pace of change is unique to each individual and requires patience, persistence, and understanding. Setbacks may occur, but they are part of the healing process. Therapists should celebrate small victories and reinforce the progress made, even if it seems incremental. Supportive feedback and encouragement strengthen the therapeutic relationship and boost patients' confidence in their capacity to change.

Lastly, healthcare professionals need to foster an environment that supports ongoing learning and adaptation. Continuous education on emerging evidence and therapeutic approaches is vital for improving patient outcomes. Sharing knowledge and experiences within a network of colleagues can enhance collective expertise and innovation in trauma therapy, ensuring that belief systems are approached with the nuance and depth they deserve.

In summary, belief systems influenced by trauma serve as both challenges and opportunities within cognitive theory. By understanding and addressing these systems, mental health professionals can help individuals redefine their relationships with trauma, paving the way for healing and transformation.

Understanding Thought Patterns

In the intricate web of trauma therapy, understanding thought patterns is not just valuable—it's pivotal. As we delve deeper into cognitive theory, we encounter the mental scripts and narratives individuals develop after traumatic experiences. These thought patterns can often dictate the trajectory of a person's mental health, influencing their emotions and reactions. So, why focus on understanding thought patterns? It's because these patterns can either imprison survivors in a cycle of distress or liberate them as they move towards healing.

Thought patterns are the mental frameworks that shape how individuals interpret their world and experiences. For those who have endured trauma, these patterns often become skewed, resulting in negative or maladaptive beliefs. This is where cognitive theory plays a crucial role. By examining these cognitive distortions, mental health professionals can assist individuals in identifying and rectifying harmful thoughts, ultimately guiding them toward a pathway of cognitive clarity and emotional resilience.

The impact of trauma frequently leads to all-or-nothing thinking, overgeneralization, and catastrophic thinking, among other patterns. For instance, a person who has experienced a traumatic event might believe that they're powerless or that the world is unsafe, even when such perceptions don't align with reality. These thought patterns are not mere reflections but distortions that persist, creating barriers to recovery. By bringing these distortions into awareness, practitioners open the door to cognitive restructuring and healing.

The therapeutic process necessitates a journey into these thought patterns. This journey involves identifying the automatic thoughts that surface in response to triggering stimuli. For those affected by trauma, these automatic thoughts might be self-critical and blame-oriented, contributing to a cycle of self-doubt and shame. The task of therapists is to help individuals challenge these automatic responses and, through cognitive therapy techniques, replace them with more balanced and constructive narratives.

One of the essential aspects of cognitive theory in trauma treatment is how it frames these thought patterns as neither permanent nor unchangeable. By doing so, it empowers both therapists and clients with the optimism that transformation is attainable. Establishing this foundation is critical, as it fosters an environment where change is not just a distant hope but an achievable reality. Through collaborative efforts, the therapeutic alliance becomes a crucible for reconstructing thought patterns that were once perceived as immutable.

Research has consistently shown that cognitive restructuring—the process of shifting maladaptive thought patterns—is vital in alleviating symptoms of PTSD and other trauma-related disorders. The evidence suggests that when individuals reshape their thoughts, they gain greater control over their emotional responses and behaviors. This empowering process promotes resilience and aids in breaking free from the shackles of past trauma.

However, understanding thought patterns can't be limited to recognizing distortions. It involves appreciating the context in which these patterns developed—the socio-cultural and environmental factors that interact with individual cognitions. The acknowledgment of such influences enables a more nuanced and sophisticated approach to therapy, one that honors the complexity of each person's narrative and lived experience.

For health care providers, researchers, and mental health professionals, blending cognitive theory with trauma understanding requires a delicate balance of empathy and skill. Effective intervention hinges on their ability to not only identify thought patterns but also to foster an empathetic environment where clients feel safe to explore their cognitive landscapes. This involves being attuned to subtle cues and open to the multiplicity of each person's experience.

Graduate students and trainees entering this field should be aware of the profound impact thought patterns have on treatment outcomes. As burgeoning professionals, their engagement in this process is key to mastering the art and science of trauma therapy. They must cultivate an awareness and sensitivity towards how thought patterns are articulated and their subsequent influence on a client's outlook and actions.

In advancing the practice of understanding thought patterns, clinical supervisors and educators serve as torchbearers, guiding the next generation. They play a pivotal role in instilling a deep comprehension of cognitive theory and its application in trauma therapy. By doing so, they equip practitioners with tools to evolve continually, promoting an ethos of compassionate care and evidence-based practice.

Ultimately, the goal is to reclaim mental space and foster healing in those affected by trauma. By dissecting and reconstructing thought patterns, therapists and clients collaboratively rewrite narratives. This rewriting not only paves the way for cognitive and emotional liberation but also allows for a reinvigorated sense of agency and hope.

Influenced by the intricacies of human cognition, the understanding of thought patterns remains at the heart of transforming therapeutic practices. It underscores the shared journey of healing, affirming that while trauma may alter the architecture of our thoughts, with intention and guidance, these patterns can be rewoven into a fabric of resilience and strength. In this transformative process, we find not only therapeutic success but also a profound testament to the resilience of the human spirit.

CHAPTER
5

INTRODUCTION TO CPT SESSIONS

Diving into the heart of Cognitive Processing Therapy (CPT) begins with understanding the essence of its sessions. Each CPT session offers a structured sanctuary where healing unfolds, guiding both therapist and patient toward transformative breakthroughs.

Within these environments, therapists step into a dual role as educators and compassionate guides, skillfully fostering a space that beckons engagement and dynamic participation. The rhythms of these sessions are designed to empower patients, encouraging them to confront and reconstruct their narratives of trauma with newfound clarity. This collaborative journey doesn't just shift thought patterns; it builds a foundation of resilience, engaging the patient's intrinsic strengths in ways that inspire and renew. As sessions unfold, the therapeutic alliance—carved out through empathy and expert guidance becomes a beacon illuminating the path to reclaiming one's mental fortitude and peace, setting the stage for profound personal growth and healing.

Structure of Sessions

Understanding the structure of CPT sessions is akin to knowing the blueprint of a house before construction begins. Knowing the order and flow is essential, but it's crucial to remember that each therapeutic session is also a dynamic interaction between the therapist and the patient. This structure not only guides the therapist but also offers the patient a sense of predictability and safety, crucial for individuals navigating the turbulent waters of trauma.

Typically, sessions in Cognitive Processing Therapy are structured to follow a consistent pattern. Each session serves a distinct purpose in the therapeutic journey. While there's flexibility to tailor to specific needs, generally sessions begin with a brief review of the previous session, highlighting key insights or breakthroughs. This orientation helps in maintaining continuity and keeping the therapeutic goals in focus.

Following this review, the session usually transitions into a discussion of any practice assignments the patient was asked to complete. These assignments are more than just tasks; they're vital components that help patients integrate new perspectives into their daily lives. Feedback on these assignments is imperative. It's not merely about whether the task was completed but about what the process revealed to the patient and how it felt. This phase is often rich with insights into the patient's progress.

As the session progresses, introducing new content or therapeutic exercises takes center stage. This could involve exploring specific cognitive patterns, engaging in structured activities to challenge maladaptive thoughts, or introducing new emotional processing skills. The therapist's role during this juncture is twofold: they act as both a coach and a guide, facilitating the patient's journey towards self-discovery and healing.

Sessions wrap up by discussing insights uncovered during the current meeting and reinforcing the connection between these insights and the patient's broader therapeutic goals. Additionally, setting up practice assignments for the forthcoming week keeps the momentum going. This consistency helps patients maintain an active role in their healing process, promoting a sense of autonomy and mastery over their therapeutic journey.

Within this structure, it's essential for therapists to be vigilant and responsive to the patient's emotional cues. Not every session will fit neatly into this format. There will be times when a patient may arrive with an urgent need to discuss a pressing issue. Flexibility is key, allowing for adjustments while still striving to cover the agenda by the session's conclusion, thus maintaining a sense of rhythm and progress.

Interestingly, while structure provides a roadmap, it's the therapist's empathy and ability to connect that truly fuels healing. Creating a safe and supportive environment is as crucial as the session's content. Patients often bring deeply personal and painful experiences into the session. The therapist must foster an atmosphere where such vulnerability is met with compassion and understanding, not judgment or impatience.

The sessions are iterative – one building upon the last. It's much like a spiral, where efforts may seem repetitive, but each cycle deepens patient insight and emotional processing. This repetition helps patients unlearn ingrained and unhelpful thought patterns and replace them with healthier, adaptive ones.

The heart of these sessions lies in assisting patients to uncover and challenge distorted cognitions related to their trauma. The skills developed in these sessions empower individuals to reclaim their autonomy from the grip of PTSD. As each session unfolds, patients often move from a position of viewing themselves through a lens of trauma to understanding their inherent worth and resilience.

As sessions conclude, leaving on a note of hope and reassurance can't be understated. Whether through affirmations, encouragement about patient progress, or simply a reminder of their innate strength, these positive closures play a profound role in sustaining patient engagement throughout the treatment.

The structure of CPT sessions, therefore, is not just a series of therapeutic checkpoints but a carefully curated pathway leading to restoration and empowerment. It combines evidence-based strategies with compassion and flexibility, allowing for a holistic approach to healing. For mental health providers, being adept in this structure means being equipped not only with tools for intervention but also with the empathy necessary for true therapeutic connection. This strategic and empathetic framework ultimately helps in unlocking the transformative potential inherent in each session.

Therapist's Role

In the intricate dance of cognitive processing therapy (CPT), the therapist plays a pivotal role, guiding the rhythm and flow of sessions. Like a seasoned conductor leading an orchestra, the therapist ensures that each component of the therapy process harmonizes to foster healing. Understanding the complexity of trauma and its ripple effects on cognition and emotion, therapists are tasked with creating a therapeutic environment where trust and exploratory courage bloom.

Therapists must wear multiple hats throughout CPT sessions. At the heart of their role is the creation of a supportive atmosphere where clients feel safe enough to explore painful memories and emotions. This setting is fundamental not only to engage clients but also to encourage the honest sharing that is essential for effective therapy. A therapist's emotional intelligence is a powerful tool here, allowing them to attune to the client's needs and adjust the session's tempo accordingly.

Educating clients about PTSD and the cognitive processes involved is another critical aspect of the therapist's role. This involves communicating complex psychological concepts in digestible language, empowering clients with knowledge about how trauma affects their thoughts and beliefs. By fostering an understanding of the cognitive distortions that may arise post-trauma, therapists help clients reclaim agency over their thoughts and begin the transformative process of cognitive restructuring.

Moreover, therapists act as guides through the challenging terrain of thought records and trauma narratives, helping clients to articulate and examine their experiences. This guidance is not merely instructional; it's inspirational, mirroring the therapists' belief in the client's capacity for change. In doing so, therapists provide scaffolding for clients as they confront and amend distorted thoughts, paving the way for healthier cognitive patterns.

Listening is an equally vital skill for therapists, one that underpins the therapeutic alliance. Active listening does not just involve hearing the words but understanding the emotions and beliefs interwoven within them. This empathetic engagement fosters trust, making the therapist a confidant and a catalyst for meaningful change. Listening involves capturing nuances in the client's speech, acknowledging both spoken and unspoken fears, and reflecting back deep understanding and acceptance.

Therapists also need to be adept at managing emotional intensity, both in themselves and their clients. Sessions often bring latent emotions to the surface, requiring therapists to remain grounded and regulated. This stability provides a model for clients, demonstrating how they might manage their emotional responses outside the therapy room. The therapist's calm presence acts as an anchor for clients in the stormy sea of emotion, offering a sense of safety and reassurance.

Throughout the therapeutic journey, therapists balance structure with flexibility. While they follow a structured approach to ensure that sessions cover necessary topics and interventions, they must also remain attuned to the client's pace and adapt as needed. This might involve adjusting the session plan if a client is not ready to tackle a particular issue or feels overwhelmed. The ability to pivot and respond to the client's immediate needs is critical in maintaining a supportive and effective therapeutic alliance.

Additionally, therapists serve as role models of resilience and hope. They embody the principles they teach, demonstrating a commitment to ongoing learning, self-care, and personal growth. By sharing appropriate parts of their own journey (when suitable) and showing vulnerability, they instill confidence in the client's ability to overcome challenges. They remind clients that progress, albeit sometimes slow, is attainable through perseverance and effort.

The mentorship aspect of the therapist's role is particularly significant when working with clients from diverse backgrounds or those with complex trauma histories. Understanding cultural nuances and showing respect for the client's unique worldview enhances therapeutic rapport. This cultural humility allows therapists to tailor their approach, ensuring the therapy is accessible and relevant to the client's lived experience.

Another facet of the therapist's role is the continuous assessment of progress, which involves a dance of observation, questioning, and feedback collection. Through regular check-ins, therapists can gauge the efficacy of interventions and make necessary adjustments. They invite clients to reflect on shifts in their thinking and behavior, reinforcing achievements and sustaining motivation. Encouraging self-reflection strengthens the client's self-awareness and helps solidify new cognitive patterns.

Ultimately, the therapist's role in CPT is a dynamic, multifaceted endeavor. It demands a blend of skills and qualities, including empathy, adaptability, and fortitude. By skillfully combining these elements, therapists guide their clients toward recovery, empowering them to reclaim not only their mental processes but also their lives. In doing so, they fulfill the profound and rewarding mission of facilitating healing while fostering hope and resilience. Through this partnership, therapists and clients together illuminate the path from trauma to empowerment, reflecting the transformative essence of cognitive processing therapy itself.

Patient Engagement Strategies

Every therapeutic journey begins with embarking on a pathway that places patient engagement at its core. Especially within the framework of Cognitive Processing Therapy (CPT), engaging patients isn't just an initial hurdle—it's a continuous endeavor that threads through the entirety of the therapy. Entrusting patients with an active role in their healing process enriches their ability to navigate a transformative experience. But how exactly do we foster such meaningful engagement?

Firstly, respecting the patient's unique story is paramount. Each individual bringing their trauma to CPT sessions has lived a narrative that defies simplistic categorization. It's crucial for practitioners to communicate that these sessions are a collaborative space where their experiences are not just acknowledged but deeply understood. This approach contributes to cultivating a safe and empowering environment, laying a foundation where genuine engagement can flourish.

Listening actively goes beyond hearing words; it's about grasping the nuances and emotions woven into those words. When patients perceive a therapist's genuine interest, they are more likely to engage and invest in the therapeutic process. Active listening, hence, is not a passive act but rather an exchange that encourages more profound reflections and contributions from patients. Such interactions build trust and make the patients feel seen and valued.

Moreover, incorporating psychoeducation as part of engagement strategies pivots around making knowledge accessible and relatable. When patients understand the workings of PTSD and the cognitive processes involved, it demystifies the therapy. An informed patient is better positioned to engage with the therapeutic techniques consciously and intentionally, as they comprehend the rationale behind each session's structure.

In any therapeutic setting, addressing patients' concerns—be they about the therapy process or their life circumstances—shouldn't be an afterthought. Validating these concerns and integrating them into the therapeutic strategy can empower patients, making them feel more in control and involved. While therapists guide the journey, true engagement arises when patients feel their struggles and aspirations are steering the direction.

The setting of therapy goals isn't merely administrative; it's a mutual contract of sorts, establishing accountability. These goals should arise from a dialogue where patients express their hopes and therapists translate these into practical steps. By involving patients in this goal-setting phase, they invest emotionally in the outcomes, making them active participants rather than passive recipients.

Innovatively, engaging with technology, when applicable, could be an ally in patient engagement strategies. Some patients may find solace in digital tracking of their thoughts or listening to mindfulness exercises outside sessions. Introducing such tools enables patients to engage with therapy even beyond the physical confines of the therapist's office.

Nevertheless, potential barriers to engagement should be anticipated and discussed openly. Whether it's ambivalence, past negative experiences with therapy, or a general mistrust of clinical interventions, these issues deserve space within the therapeutic dialogue. Addressing them candidly can prevent them from becoming hindrances and, instead, transform these barriers into bridges of understanding and empathy.

One can't overlook cultural sensitivity and adaptability when engaging patients from diverse backgrounds. Each cultural backdrop harbors unique perceptions of mental health and wellness. A nuanced understanding and respectful acknowledgment of these cultural nuances ensure that patients don't feel alienated by a one-size-fits-all approach. Instead, they can see themselves in the therapeutic process, thus enhancing their willingness to engage.

The role of self-reflection as a tool for patient engagement is often underestimated. Encouraging patients to reflect not only on their progress but also on their emotional responses to therapy can heighten their awareness and commitment. Self-reflection aligns beautifully with the principles of cognitive therapy, enhancing a continual introspection that's critical for long-lasting transformation.

Ultimately, the art of patient engagement within CPT sessions is a choreography of empathy, adaptability, and respect. It's about coaxing forth the patient's intrinsic motivations and aligning them with therapeutic rigor. Through this intricate dance, therapists and patients weave together a tapestry of healing, one that respects the complexity of trauma while nurturing the profound capacity for recovery.

CHAPTER 6

BUILDING THERAPEUTIC ALLIANCE

In the journey of healing from trauma, the therapeutic alliance serves as the cornerstone for meaningful progress. It's not only about applying techniques, but about creating a partnership rooted in trust and empathy. This relationship empowers patients and clinicians alike, facilitating an open and honest exchange that paves the way for transformative change. Effective communication is the key; it requires active listening, genuine understanding, and timely compassion. Clinicians must be attuned to their patients' words and silences, signals that offer invaluable insights beyond spoken narratives. Trust can be fragile, but it's strengthened by maintaining professional boundaries that instill a sense of safety and respect. This alliance is more than a clinical relationship; it's a collaborative journey towards healing that honors the resilience and vulnerability of the individuals we serve. In fostering this connection, we not only guide patients through the complexities of trauma but also offer them a space where they can reclaim their time and mental peace, step by step.

The therapeutic alliance is truly a dynamic, evolving relationship that goes beyond the traditional roles of therapist and patient. Research has shown that the quality of this relationship can significantly impact the outcome of trauma therapy, with studies suggesting that the stronger the therapeutic alliance, the better the likelihood of achieving positive results. This connection doesn't happen overnight; it takes time to establish and requires patience, consistency, and empathy from the clinician. One of the most powerful aspects of the therapeutic alliance is the sense of validation it provides. When individuals feel heard and understood in their most vulnerable states, it can be a deeply healing experience, especially for those who have been silenced or marginalized due to their trauma. This validation is crucial in helping patients rebuild their sense of self-worth and trust in others, which are often severely damaged by trauma.

Over time, this alliance fosters a collaborative environment where patients are not just passive recipients of therapy but active participants in their own healing process.

An often overlooked but essential aspect of the therapeutic alliance is the clinician's own awareness of their biases, emotions, and limitations. Trauma work can be intense, and clinicians must be mindful of their emotional reactions and ensure they do not inadvertently impose their perspectives onto the patient. Reflective supervision and ongoing professional development play vital roles in helping clinicians maintain their capacity for empathy and effectiveness. This level of self-awareness allows therapists to remain attuned to the evolving needs of their patients while also ensuring they maintain a healthy professional distance, which is necessary for preserving both the integrity of the therapeutic relationship and their own well-being. Interestingly, studies suggest that clinicians who engage in their own self-care and seek support for their emotional responses to trauma work tend to be more effective in their practice, as they are able to remain present and emotionally available for their patients without becoming overwhelmed by the emotional weight of the work. Ultimately, a balanced, thoughtful therapeutic alliance not only empowers the patient but also supports the clinician in providing the most compassionate and effective care possible.

Communication Skills

In the journey of building a therapeutic alliance, communication skills stand as the cornerstone. The power of effective communication lies not just in what is said, but how it's conveyed and interpreted. It's about creating a space where patients feel seen, heard, and understood. This connection allows therapists to delve deeper, forging a relationship built on mutual trust and respect.

The first step in honing communication skills is active listening. Active listening goes beyond merely hearing words; it means being fully present and engaged. This involves pausing internal dialogue to truly absorb the patient's words and emotions. Therapists must respond with empathy, reflecting understanding both verbally and nonverbally. When a patient senses they are genuinely being listened to, it fosters a safe environment conducive to healing.

Nonverbal cues are equally critical in communication. Therapists use body language, eye contact, and facial expressions to communicate empathy and understanding. These subtle signals can significantly affect the therapeutic alliance, sometimes more profoundly than words themselves. A warm smile, a slight nod, or a calm demeanor can reassure patients and encourage them to open up further.

It's essential to tailor communication to the individual's unique needs and cultural context. Every patient has distinct experiences that shape their perspective. Effective communication requires sensitivity to cultural nuances and variations in communication styles. This involves therapists being aware of their own biases and maintaining an open-minded approach.

Establishing a rapport with patients is vital for effective communication. Rapport serves as the bridge over which trust traverses. Building rapport involves demonstrating genuine interest and commitment to the patient's well-being. By sharing small personal anecdotes or maintaining a onversational tone, therapists humanize themselves, making the professional relationship less intimidating.

A critical aspect of therapeutic communication is feedback, which should be constructive and supportive. Providing feedback involves balancing validation with gentle challenges to their cognitive and emotional processes. This balanced approach motivates patients to reflect on their thoughts and behaviors without feeling judged or dismissed.

Empathetic communication also requires patience and the ability to tolerate silence. Silence can be uncomfortable, but it often presents opportunities for introspective thinking. It allows patients to process their emotions and thoughts at their own pace. Therapists who can sit comfortably in silence often find that it provokes deeper insight and self-awareness in their patients.

Furthermore, clear and concise language is necessary to avoid misunderstandings. Complex psychological jargon can confuse or alienate patients, erecting barriers to understanding. Therapists should strive to simplify explanations and use analogies that are relatable, ensuring information is digestible and applicable.

As therapists navigate the intricacies of communication, they must also maintain professional boundaries. Clear boundaries create a framework within which professional relationships can flourish healthily. Being too informal might jeopardize the therapeutic space, while being overly rigid could stifle open communication. Finding the right balance is key.

Humor, used appropriately, can also be a valuable communication tool. It can diffuse tension and help patients view their situations from a new perspective. However, it's crucial to gauge the patient's comfort level with humor, ensuring it's inclusive and supportive rather than dismissive or mocking.

Effective communication isn't just a single skill but a tapestry of strategies that require constant practice and refinement. Therapists must remain committed to developing these skills through ongoing education and supervision. They should seek feedback from peers and mentors, using it as a catalyst for professional growth.

Finally, it's important to remember that communication is a two-way street. Therapists should encourage patients to express any discomfort or misunderstanding. This openness fosters an environment where patients feel empowered to communicate their needs, enhancing their engagement and investment in the therapeutic process.

In the grand scheme of therapy, communication acts as the heartbeat of the therapeutic alliance. It facilitates understanding, nurtures trust, and ultimately empowers patients to reclaim control over their lives. By continuously striving to enhance these skills, therapists can unlock the full potential of the transformative journey their patients undertake.

Establishing Trust

Establishing trust within a therapeutic setting is both an art and a science. It's the cornerstone of the therapeutic alliance, acting as a bridge between the therapist and the patient. Without trust, even the most scientifically grounded therapeutic techniques can falter, leaving patients feeling misunderstood and unsupported. But with trust, a safe space is created where healing can truly begin. This trust is cultivated through a combination of consistent communication, empathy, and reliability.

Trust-building begins with the therapist's ability to listen genuinely. By fully attending to a patient's narrative without interruption, clinicians send a powerful message: the patient's experiences and feelings are valued and heard. This approach not only provides affirmation but also grants space for patients to recount their experiences at their own pace. It's essential that therapists resist the urge to prematurely analyze or offer solutions; often, just being present and affirming is enough to foster trust in the early stages of therapy.

Equally crucial is the therapist's capacity to convey empathy. Empathy serves as the connective tissue in therapeutic relationships, allowing patients to feel understood at a deeper level. Therapists can express empathy both verbally and nonverbally, through body language, eye contact, and reflective listening. It's the genuine connection to their patients' emotions that builds relational depth and authenticity. This process is about walking alongside the patient, acknowledging their pain, and showing commitment to their healing journey.

Beyond empathy and listening, transparency plays a vital role in establishing trust. Being transparent about therapy objectives, the therapeutic process, and professional boundaries can demystify therapy for patients, who might otherwise feel uncertain or apprehensive. When expectations are finely articulated and consent is sought before advancing therapeutic interventions, patient anxiety decreases and trust grows. This openness minimizes ambiguity and enhances the therapeutic connection.

Consistency and reliability solidify the trust-building framework. Regular, predictable sessions and the therapist's punctuality reinforce the idea that the therapist is dependable. This reliability extends beyond time- keeping—it's also reflected in the therapist's reactions and responses. Patients need to feel confident that their therapist can handle the full spectrum of their emotions, whether it's anger, grief, or despair. Demonstrating stability in the face of these emotions ensures that patients trust the therapist to journey with them through the complexities of their trauma.

Acknowledging and respecting boundaries is another crucial element of trust. Establishing and maintaining professional boundaries provides a structured framework within which therapy occurs. This structure helps patients feel secure, fostering an environment where they can explore difficult topics without fear of overstepping. The therapist's role in this dynamic is to guide the conversation gently back to therapeutic goals and keep the process on track, always considering the patient's readiness and comfort level.

Another challenge lies in recognizing and addressing cultural, social, and personal factors that influence the patient's worldview. Therapists must be aware of their own biases and work actively to remain culturally sensitive. Recognizing and validating the unique experiences of patients from diverse backgrounds enhances trust by showing that the therapist respects and values the patient's individual context.

Patients recovering from traumatic experiences may face unique trust barriers, due in part to past violations of that trust. Here, the therapist's role embodies a dual approach of caution and reassurance.

It's necessary to validate the patient's wariness while persistently demonstrating actions that build reliability and dependability. Trust is not obtained through grand gestures; rather, it is nurtured through consistent, small acts that demonstrate care and understanding.

Repeating affirmations and summaries of a patient's words can affirm their experiences, turning abstract feelings into tangible validations. This technique, sometimes referred to as reflective listening, doesn't just confirm what was said but demonstrates an understanding of the emotions and perspectives behind the words. Such actions can incrementally enhance a patient's willingness to open up, seeing that their therapist truly comprehends their internal world.

Over time, as trust deepens, patients will start to share more vulnerable parts of their experiences. The gentle uncovering of these layers can lead to a profound transformation within the therapeutic context, often providing a breakthrough in treatment.

However, the therapist must remain vigilant, observing not just the words but also body language and other nonverbal cues that indicate comfort or discomfort. Adjustments in approach based on these observations can make all the difference in maintaining a trusting relationship.

Ultimately, establishing trust is an ongoing process that flourishes in an environment of mutual respect, transparency, and unwavering support. It requires therapists to engage actively, mentally, and emotionally, thereby creating a therapeutic space that can hold and nurture the vulnerability and courage patients bring into the room. The development of this trust is essential for the success of any therapeutic endeavor, laying the groundwork for a transformative alliance that respects both therapist and patient as partners in the journey toward healing.

Maintaining Professional Boundaries

The cornerstone of effective therapy lies in the delicate balance between empathy and professionalism. Professional boundaries serve as a framework within which therapeutic relationships thrive. They enable therapists to create a safe, respectful environment conducive to healing. Navigating these boundaries requires not only skill but also a keen awareness of their dynamic nature. In the context of PTSD and trauma- focused therapy, upholding these boundaries becomes even more crucial.

Maintaining professional boundaries is about setting limits that protect both the therapist and the patient. This isn't about distancing oneself emotionally, but rather ensuring the therapeutic process is beneficial and ethical. Boundaries help in preventing the development of dual relationships, which could compromise the therapeutic environment. The goal is to foster a professional relationship that supports the patient's growth while preserving the therapist's objectivity.

Therapists often encounter challenges when it comes to maintaining boundaries because each therapeutic relationship is unique, presenting its own complexities. For instance, the therapist's role is inherently empathetic, potentially leading to blurred lines as they share in the patient's healing journey. However, it is paramount that therapists remain aware of their professional identity and limitations. This mindfulness helps to avoid over-identifying with the patient or becoming too emotionally involved.

One effective method of maintaining professional boundaries is through clear communication from the outset. During initial assessments, it's important that therapists explicitly outline their roles, the goals of therapy, and the rules governing their professional interactions. Patients need to understand what they can expect from the therapeutic relationship and what is expected of them. This clarity helps prevent misunderstandings and establishes a foundation of trust.

Setting boundaries doesn't mean being inflexible; rather, it's about having the wisdom to know when to adjust them to best serve the patient's needs and therapeutic process. Situations may arise that require the therapist to reconsider the boundaries in place. For instance, a patient may reach out during a crisis outside of regular hours. In such cases, therapists must weigh the benefit of being available against the risk of dependence or burnout.

Regular supervision is another critical strategy in boundary maintenance. Engaging in supervision provides therapists with an opportunity to reflect on their practice, gain insight into their relational dynamics with patients, and ensure they're adhering to ethical practices. Supervisors can provide a fresh perspective, offer guidance on managing complex situations, and support therapists in sustaining their boundaries.

Boundaries are not only about what therapists should do; they also define what therapists should not do.

Engaging in social relationships with patients, accepting extravagant gifts, or allowing therapy sessions to drift off-purpose can all compromise professional boundaries. These actions risk undermining the therapeutic process and can harm the patient's progress. Therapists must be vigilant in recognizing these potential pitfalls and maintaining a correct course.

The concept of boundaries extends to the digital realm as well. With the increasing use of technology in therapy, including telehealth and online communication, therapists need to navigate the nuances of digital boundaries. It involves setting guidelines for online communication, ensuring confidentiality, and defining the limits of digital interactions. This aspect of boundary maintenance requires ongoing education and adaptation to new technologies.

Maintaining professional boundaries isn't a static task. It requires continuous vigilance and a commitment to ethical practice. It's essential for therapists to periodically revisit their boundaries and consult with colleagues to address any ambiguities or challenges. This can prevent boundary issues from escalating and ensure that the therapeutic alliance remains focused and constructive.

While therapists must hold themselves accountable to professional standards, it's also crucial to understand the role of self-care in maintaining effective boundaries. Self-care isn't just a personal indulgence; it's a professional necessity. Therapists who neglect their well-being may struggle to maintain clear boundaries, leading to emotional exhaustion or reduced effectiveness in their practice. Regular self-care routines help therapists remain grounded and present, allowing them to offer their best to each patient.

Boundaries, when well-maintained, enhance the therapeutic alliance by fostering a relationship built on trust, respect, and collaboration. Patients benefit from knowing they are working with a professional committed to ethical care, while therapists find satisfaction in the clarity and safety that strong boundaries provide. This mutual respect and understanding create a space where healing and recovery can truly flourish.

CHAPTER
7

EDUCATION ABOUT PTSD

Advancing the understanding of PTSD among mental health professionals is crucial for transforming clients' lives, and this chapter focuses on equipping you with the knowledge and techniques necessary to achieve that. By employing strategic psychoeducation techniques, healthcare providers can demystify PTSD, enabling clients to grasp the intricacies of their experiences. Explaining brain function in a way that's accessible helps illuminate how trauma impacts cognition and behavior, fostering a path towards healing. Furthermore, confronting and correcting prevailing misconceptions about PTSD can dismantle stigmas, leading to more empathetic and effective care. As you delve into these educational strategies, remember the goal is not just to share information, but to inspire growth, resilience, and empowerment in those you serve. Embrace this journey as a profound opportunity to facilitate deeper understanding and foster meaningful change for your clients' futures.

Psychoeducation Techniques

Psychoeducation plays a pivotal role in the treatment of PTSD and serves as a foundation for healing. Through the process of psychoeducation, individuals gain a clearer understanding of PTSD and its effects on their lives, helping them navigate the complexities of this condition with a sense of empowerment and hope. Delivering psychoeducation isn't merely about sharing information—it's about equipping individuals with the knowledge that can transform trauma into a more manageable part of their narrative.

Psychoeducation in the context of PTSD involves explaining the physiological, psychological, and behavioral symptoms of the disorder. This knowledge dispels myths and misconceptions that patients often encounter. It's crucial that health care providers communicate complex information in a digestible manner, ensuring that it resonates with each individual's personal experience. Presenting information with empathy and clarity can foster a deeper connection, enhancing the therapeutic alliance.

One of the primary techniques in psychoeducation is normalizing the wide array of emotions and reactions someone with PTSD might experience. Facilitators of this process can reassure individuals that their symptoms are a common response to trauma, not a sign of personal failure or weakness. By framing reactions such as hypervigilance, avoidance, and intrusive thoughts as normal, yet challenging, responses to trauma, individuals may begin to reframe their self-perceptions and reduce self-stigmatization.

Another key technique involves educating individuals about the brain's role in PTSD. Understanding the neurobiological impacts of trauma can help individuals grasp why they might react in certain ways and why some responses feel involuntary or overpowering. This can be achieved by explaining the functions of the amygdala, hippocampus, and prefrontal cortex in lay terms, highlighting how each part of the brain contributes to the symptoms of PTSD. When clients understand how their brain works in the context of trauma, they often feel relieved and justified in their experiences.

Clarifying misconceptions is also a critical component of psychoeducation. Many individuals hold inaccurate beliefs about PTSD, such as thinking it only affects those with combat experience, or that it's a sign of enduring psychological fragility. Addressing these misconceptions can prevent individuals from feeling isolated or misunderstood. Educators should encourage open dialogue where individuals feel safe sharing their beliefs and asking questions that may have been sources of shame or confusion.

Another effective technique is the use of metaphors and visual aids that can simplify complex concepts. Metaphors can bridge the gap between abstract scientific findings and personal experience. For instance, comparing the brain to a control center disrupted by traumatic events can help individuals visualize the impact of PTSD. Visual aids, like diagrams and flowcharts, can further reinforce these concepts, offering a visual representation that makes the information more relatable and memorable.

Interactive methods, such as group discussions and role-playing, can also enhance the psychoeducational process. In group settings, individuals have the opportunity to share experiences and learn from others facing similar challenges, fostering a sense of community and shared understanding. Role-playing can help individuals practice and internalize coping strategies in a supportive environment.

The use of storytelling is another engaging approach. By sharing narratives of those who have successfully managed PTSD, individuals can find hope and inspiration in their own journey. Stories offer relatable paths of resilience and recovery, providing concrete examples of how psychoeducation can translate into real-world change.

Psychoeducation should also focus on strategies to cope with and manage PTSD symptoms. This includes providing tools for emotional regulation, stress reduction techniques, and nurturing mindfulness practices. When clients learn these techniques, they can begin to apply them in their daily lives, fostering a sense of agency and self-efficacy.

Adapting psychoeducational techniques to the individual's unique cultural and contextual background is essential. Culturally sensitive materials show respect for diverse backgrounds and can enhance the effectiveness of psychoeducation. Tailoring information to align with cultural values and beliefs helps ensure that materials are relevant and applicable to each individual's life.

To assess the effectiveness of psychoeducation, it is helpful for providers to ask for feedback from their clients. This ongoing dialogue can guide adjustments in the approach to better meet the individual's needs. It emphasizes that learning about PTSD is an evolving process and should be customized to each person's pace and comprehension level.

Ultimately, the successful implementation of psychoeducation techniques requires commitment, empathy, and adaptability from healthcare providers. As therapists embrace these educational techniques, they equip individuals not only with knowledge but also with renewed compassion for themselves, lightening the burden of PTSD. In empowering individuals, psychoeducation transforms from simply delivering information to igniting a spark of hope—hope that enables healing and reclaiming control over one's life.

Explaining Brain Function

The human brain, with its remarkable complexity, plays a pivotal role in how individuals experience and respond to traumatic events. When discussing PTSD, it's essential to understand how brain function can be altered by trauma. Such insights not only inform therapeutic interventions but also help demystify the symptoms experienced by those with PTSD. For healthcare providers, researchers, and educators, a deep comprehension of these processes is foundational to effectively supporting patients.

The brain continually processes information, but in the context of trauma, this can lead to dysregulation within certain neural circuits. The amygdala, often referred to as the brain's "fear center," becomes hyperactive after a traumatic event. This heightened state of alertness can make individuals more sensitive to potential threats, both real and perceived. Typically, the prefrontal cortex—responsible for rational thinking and decision-making—regulates the amygdala's response. However, in individuals with PTSD, this regulation is often impaired, leading to an exaggerated stress response.

In contrast, the hippocampus, a region of the brain involved in forming new memories and distinguishing between past and present experiences, often shows reduced volume and functionality in those suffering from PTSD. This reduction can contribute to the intrusive memories and flashbacks that characterize the disorder. When the hippocampus is unable to effectively contextualize traumatic memories, individuals might experience these memories as though they are occurring in the present, rather than recollections from the past.

Understanding these brain mechanisms provides a biological basis for the symptoms of PTSD, thus underlining the importance of neuroscience in psychological therapy. It helps remove some of the stigma associated with PTSD by framing it as a physiological reaction to trauma rather than a character flaw. For mental health professionals, this knowledge also supports the development of targeted therapies aimed at promoting neurobiological healing and better emotional regulation.

Regarding therapeutic implications, interventions such as Cognitive Processing Therapy (CPT) can help in rewiring the affected neural pathways. By challenging and reframing negative thought patterns, CPT encourages the prefrontal cortex to reassert control over the amygdala, thus mitigating fear responses. Over time, such therapies can catalyze neuroplastic changes that diminish PTSD symptoms.

Moreover, the integration of mindfulness and grounding techniques in therapy can facilitate the recalibration of brain circuits. These practices encourage patients to focus on the present moment, which can reduce the amygdala's activity and, concurrently, reinforce the regulatory functions of the prefrontal cortex. By retraining the brain to remain in the present, rather than reliving the trauma, patients can achieve a sense of stability and control over their emotional responses.

The conversation about brain function and PTSD also extends into the realm of ongoing research. Fields like neuroimaging have advanced our understanding by visualizing changes in brain activity associated with PTSD. For clinicians and researchers, staying abreast of such developments is crucial. It empowers them to incorporate evidence-based practices and utilize innovations in therapy that emerge from a growing body of scientific knowledge.

Collaboration across disciplines further enriches this landscape. Neuroscientists, psychologists, and clinicians working together can create more holistic treatment approaches that address both the psychological and biological dimensions of PTSD. The future of PTSD therapy is not just about psychological discourse but about encompassing a multidimensional understanding that marries the mind and brain.

In conclusion, explaining brain function in relation to PTSD serves as a critical bridge between complex biological processes and therapeutic practice. Recognizing the interplay of brain regions in the aftermath of trauma highlights the profound impact of PTSD and advances our strategies for alleviating its distressing symptoms. For those dedicated to the field of mental health, integrating this knowledge into therapy is not just an option—it's essential.

The collaboration between neuroscientists, psychologists, and clinicians represents a paradigm shift in the way we approach trauma recovery. By merging insights from neurobiology with psychological and therapeutic strategies, a more comprehensive treatment framework is emerging. Neuroscientific research has revealed the intricate ways in which trauma impacts brain structures like the hippocampus, amygdala, and prefrontal cortex, areas responsible for memory, emotional regulation, and executive function. Understanding these biological processes allows therapists to better tailor interventions, such as Cognitive Processing Therapy (CPT) or Eye Movement Desensitization and Reprocessing (EMDR), to target not just the psychological symptoms of PTSD, but also the neurobiological factors contributing to them. For example, neurofeedback, a technique that helps train brainwaves, is becoming increasingly popular as a complementary treatment for PTSD, demonstrating that brain activity can be modified to reduce trauma-related symptoms. This integration of approaches promises to enhance therapeutic outcomes and provide a more holistic healing experience for patients.

Moreover, as the field of PTSD therapy continues to evolve, the future holds exciting possibilities for incorporating cutting-edge technologies and a deeper understanding of brain function into treatment protocols. Functional magnetic resonance imaging (fMRI) and positron emission tomography (PET) scans are now commonly used to study brain activity in real-time, allowing researchers to map how different brain regions respond to trauma-related stimuli and therapeutic interventions. This knowledge is crucial for developing personalized treatment plans that are tailored not only to an individual's trauma history but also to their specific brain function and neural responses. By combining traditional psychotherapy with newer, technology-driven approaches, clinicians are better equipped to support patients in their healing journey. As we continue to explore the complex relationship between the mind and brain, the future of PTSD therapy will likely see even more advanced, integrative methods that allow for a truly multidimensional approach to recovery, ensuring that both the biological and psychological dimensions of trauma are addressed in a compassionate, scientifically grounded manner.

Addressing Misconceptions

Misunderstandings about PTSD—Post Traumatic Stress Disorder—are as pervasive as they are problematic, not only impeding effective treatment but also adversely affecting social support systems for those affected. As mental health professionals, our role in dispelling these myths is integral to fostering an informed community and effective care.

One common misconception is that PTSD only impacts military veterans. While it's true that combat exposure can lead to PTSD, this condition is not exclusive to those in military service. PTSD affects people from all walks of life, including survivors of sexual assault, accidents, natural disasters, and various other traumatic events. Broadening the scope of who can experience PTSD helps reduce stigma and enhances access to care for countless individuals who might otherwise go unnoticed.

Another pervasive myth is the notion that PTSD manifests immediately after a traumatic incident. Contrary to this, symptoms can often surface months or even years later, complicating the diagnosis and understanding by affected individuals and their families. This delayed onset can lead to self-blame or mislabeling of behaviors and emotions, which is why education on the varied timelines of symptom emergence is crucial.

It's also vital to address the misconception that people with PTSD are permanently "damaged" or "broken". This narrative serves only to deepen the isolation and hopelessness that can accompany the disorder. Instead, it's essential to emphasize the resilience and recovery that are possible with proper treatment. Cognitive Processing Therapy (CPT), as well as other effective modalities, can significantly alleviate symptoms, leading individuals towards meaningful lives.

Moreover, it's essential to dispel the myth that individuals with PTSD are 'crazy' or unstable. Such stigmatizing language creates barriers to seeking help and can worsen outcomes by promoting fear and misunderstanding. Training on the neurobiological impacts of trauma can aid in reframing PTSD as a treatable condition rather than a character flaw or personal failing.

There's also a tendency to believe that only those with "weak" personalities develop PTSD, whereas those who are "strong" do not. Nothing could be further from the truth. The onset of PTSD is not a measure of personal fortitude but rather a complex interplay of genetics, neurobiology, and environmental factors. Educating patients and the public about this can mitigate the shame and guilt often experienced by those suffering, paving the way for more compassionate support.

Lastly, addressing misconceptions about treatment is paramount. Some believe that therapy means "reliving" the trauma, which can cause understandable apprehension. However, therapies like CPT equip individuals with tools to process and reframe traumatic experiences safely. Stressing that therapy involves more than recounting trauma—and includes understanding thoughts, feelings, and bodily responses—can encourage engagement and trust in therapeutic processes.

Addressing misconceptions isn't just about correcting false beliefs—it's about building a foundation of trust and understanding, essential components in healing. As professionals entrusted with this task, we must prioritize empathy, education, and clear communication to dismantle barriers that impede the path to recovery. By creating an accurate awareness of PTSD, we lay the groundwork for empowering our patients and reclaiming their mental health journey.

These efforts must extend beyond the clinical setting. Public education campaigns, informed discussions with policymakers, and outreach initiatives are critical to transforming misconceptions into informed perspectives. It's a collective responsibility—one where mental health education takes center stage in communities, schools, and workplaces, effectively redefining how PTSD is perceived and treated.

Ultimately, addressing misconceptions about PTSD is an ongoing endeavor. It's a commitment to continual education, reflection, and adaptation to new research and understandings. And every step taken to correct these misunderstandings brings us closer to a world where individuals affected by PTSD can access the care, respect, and support they deserve.

Expanding mental health education to include PTSD awareness in communities, schools, and workplaces is not only essential but transformative. In the workplace, for instance, research shows that when employers provide training about mental health, including PTSD, employees are more likely to seek help and experience a more supportive work environment. This proactive approach reduces stigma and fosters understanding among coworkers, ultimately enhancing productivity and job satisfaction. Schools are another critical venue where early education about mental health can significantly alter the trajectory of future generations. By teaching children and adolescents about the psychological and biological aspects of trauma, as well as how to seek help, we equip them with the tools to better understand themselves and others. Community outreach initiatives can also address systemic barriers to care, such as lack of access to mental health services or cultural stigmas, by bringing vital resources directly to those who need them. These collective efforts not only improve individual lives but also contribute to healthier, more resilient communities.

Public education campaigns and conversations with policymakers can create the groundwork for more inclusive and progressive policies that ensure PTSD care is available to everyone who needs it. Legislative efforts such as expanded access to mental health services and funding for trauma research are crucial to addressing the societal impacts of PTSD. For example, recent initiatives like the "Mental Health Parity and Addiction Equity Act" have worked to ensure that mental health treatment is covered on equal footing with physical health care, making therapy and resources more accessible. As our understanding of PTSD evolves, it is vital that our public policies do as well, adapting to the latest research and findings to provide the most effective care. Each effort to challenge misconceptions and improve public awareness contributes to a societal shift that not only changes the way PTSD is treated but also fundamentally alters how individuals living with trauma are seen and supported in every aspect of their lives. By prioritizing education and advocacy, we move closer to a future where no one affected by PTSD is left behind.

CHAPTER
8

IDENTIFYING AND CHALLENGING THOUGHTS

In the journey of cognitive processing therapy, one crucial juncture is learning to identify and challenge the thoughts that skew perception and perpetuate distress. For healthcare providers and mental health professionals, this involves guiding individuals through the process of recognizing maladaptive thoughts that may surface with alarming frequency. It's not just about pinpointing these distortions but actively engaging in cognitive restructuring techniques that allow for a reframe of these thoughts. This dynamic shift can facilitate profound changes in emotional responses and behaviors.

As professionals, the use of thought records becomes a vital tool; documenting patterns helps clients dissect and understand their thoughts in a structured way, offering a roadmap for transformation. Empowering clients to challenge these thoughts can lead to reclaiming mental space, granting a renewed sense of control and clarity. This work is imperative, as it fosters resilience and a healthier narrative, ultimately illuminating paths toward healing and growth.

The use of thought records goes beyond simply identifying negative thoughts; it offers clients a clear structure for understanding the relationship between their thoughts, emotions, and behaviors. By writing down their thoughts in real-time, individuals gain insight into the automatic cognitive processes that influence their emotional responses. This process, rooted in cognitive behavioral therapy (CBT), helps clients recognize cognitive distortions such as overgeneralization, catastrophizing, and all-or-nothing thinking, which often fuel the persistence of PTSD symptoms. Studies have shown that clients who consistently use thought records experience greater reductions in PTSD symptoms, as they are able to break the cycle of distressing thoughts and reframe them with healthier, more balanced perspectives. By making this process habitual, clients begin to cultivate a new way of thinking that can shift their overall outlook and approach to life's challenges.

In addition to improving cognitive patterns, thought records serve as a valuable tool for tracking progress over time. As clients record their thoughts and analyze the changes in their emotional reactions, they develop a greater sense of self-awareness and empowerment. This increased understanding can lead to enhanced self-efficacy, as clients witness firsthand their ability to influence their emotional state by challenging maladaptive thoughts. Furthermore, this practice fosters a sense of agency and personal growth, as individuals recognize that they are not defined by their trauma but by their capacity to learn, adapt, and heal. Research has also found that using thought records can reduce symptoms of depression and anxiety, common comorbidities of PTSD, making it a multifaceted tool in the recovery process. As clients gain more control over their thoughts and emotions, they ultimately reclaim their mental space, allowing them to move forward with greater clarity, resilience, and confidence.

Recognizing Maladaptive Thoughts

In the intricate landscape of post-traumatic stress disorder (PTSD) treatment, recognizing maladaptive thoughts emerges as a pivotal task. It's a process that demands both rigor and empathy, as therapists guide patients in identifying those thoughts that fuel distress and hinder healing. This section delves into the strategies and insights necessary for effectively recognizing these patterns, paving the way for meaningful therapeutic progress.

Maladaptive thoughts can be insidious, creeping into daily life and shaping perceptions in ways that are often detrimental. They may manifest as persistent, self-critical narratives or exaggerated fears that distort reality. Understanding these thoughts requires a nuanced approach, blending scientific inquiry with compassionate listening. Recognizing these thoughts isn't just about identifying negative patterns but understanding the context in which they occur and why they persist.

One widely effective strategy involves distinguishing between automatic and deliberate thoughts. Automatic thoughts often arise spontaneously and reflexively in response to triggers, typically without conscious awareness. In contrast, deliberate thoughts involve more cognitive processing. Encouraging patients to bring these automatic thoughts into conscious recognition allows for the critical examination necessary to challenge and alter those thoughts.

Imagine a river—thoughts have worn pathways through the mental landscape much like water carving its way through earth. Maladaptive thoughts, akin to a river diverting from its course, erode mental well- being by persistently undermining confidence and security. Clinicians are tasked with helping patients map these diversions, recognizing where and how the flow might be redirected towards healthier, constructive channels.

Cognitive models offer valuable tools in this recognition process. Using tools such as thought records, therapists can help patients capture their thoughts as they emerge in real time. This not only increases awareness but also provides a record that can be analyzed for recurring patterns. Through this method, individuals can begin to see the influence of certain thoughts on their emotions and behaviors, facilitating a deeper understanding of their impact.

At the core of recognizing maladaptive thoughts lies the idea that these thoughts are not inherently the problem; rather, it's their distortion and the influence they hold over an individual's emotional and behavioral responses. The distinction between belief and truth is crucial. Practitioners encourage patients to become curious about their thoughts—to question their validity and explore alternative perspectives that might hold more truth.

Empathy plays a decisive role in this process. Therapists must guide patients without judgment, allowing space for vulnerability and honesty. Patients must feel seen and heard, for it is within this safe therapeutic relationship that maladaptive thoughts can be acknowledged and addressed. Here, empathy acts not just as a healer but as a catalyst for change, as patients gain the courage to confront and reshape entrenched narratives.

It's also vital to consider the neurobiological underpinnings of maladaptive thinking. PTSD can alter brain function, making the recognition of thought patterns especially challenging. Understanding these biological factors can inform therapeutic approaches, emphasizing the importance of patience and persistence. This knowledge also serves to validate the experiences of those who feel their thoughts are beyond their control, fostering a non-blaming environment for exploration and growth.

Therapists often employ socratic questioning techniques to facilitate insight. By gently probing and encouraging self-reflection, patients are guided to discover discrepancies between their thoughts and objective reality. This process of guided discovery empowers individuals to independently challenge and modify their thoughts, promoting long-term cognitive resilience and adaptability.

Recognizing maladaptive thoughts is a journey towards reclaiming autonomy. Patients learn that while their thoughts have power, they themselves hold the key to change. This process cultivates a sense of agency, fostering hope and opening the door to new possibilities for healing. In taking control of their mental narratives, individuals can navigate their lives with greater peace and clarity.

It's crucial for therapists to remember that recognizing maladaptive thoughts is not an isolated task but an integral part of the therapeutic journey. This recognition is a stepping stone to subsequent strategies— cognitive restructuring and emotional processing—which further cement the foundations for sustainable, positive change. As therapists continue to guide and support, they pave the way for patients to reclaim their mental space, leading to enriched and empowered lives.

Cognitive Restructuring Techniques

Cognitive restructuring is a pivotal technique within the practice of Cognitive Processing Therapy (CPT) that empowers individuals to identify and challenge harmful or inaccurate thoughts related to trauma. This section specifically focuses on cognitive restructuring techniques that are designed to provide mental health professionals with the tools necessary to guide clients through the intricate process of transforming maladaptive thoughts. With the goal of easing the suffering caused by post-traumatic stress disorder (PTSD), these techniques foster resilience and encourage psychological growth.

The essence of cognitive restructuring lies in helping clients recognize and challenge the automatic thoughts and beliefs that intrude their daily lives, often in insidious ways. These thoughts might be rooted in trauma and can heighten distress. As a healthcare provider, the key to facilitating this shift involves not only identifying these thoughts but also helping clients reframe them in a way that is less damaging and more aligned with reality. This process encourages autonomy and builds the client's capacity to handle similar challenges in the future.

Begin with psychoeducation, which serves as the cornerstone of cognitive restructuring. Educate clients on how thoughts are not often truths. Thoughts can be misleading, distorted, or exaggerated, especially when they stem from traumatic experiences. This educational foundation lays the groundwork for clients to be active participants in their cognitive evolution. In practice, explaining the nuances of thought patterns is pivotal. An understanding of this cognitive interplay can significantly lower resistance and foster engagement in the therapeutic process.

Once clients are aware of their thought patterns, the use of thought records comes into play. Thought records are tools that help individuals document and examine their thoughts, feelings, and reactions to various stimuli. For mental health professionals, guiding clients through the structured process of recording their thoughts can illuminate the triggers and consequences of their cognitive patterns. The objective here isn't just about recording but synthesizing this information into actionable insights. Through this practice, clients can progressively uncover connections between their cognitive responses and their emotional states.

Engaging clients to challenge these thoughts, a crucial step follows. By questioning the validity of their thoughts, clients can begin to dismantle the cognitive barriers preventing their recovery. Encourage clients to ask, "Is there evidence for this thought? Is this thought a cognitive distortion?" This interrogation can help break the grip of negative or inaccurate beliefs. It's imperative that this process is handled with care and empathy, as challenging entrenched thoughts can be a vulnerable experience for the client.

Use Socratic questioning as a primary method of guiding clients through cognitive restructuring. This conversational technique, which involves a series of guiding questions, helps clients arrive at their own conclusions. Just as importantly, it fosters empowerment and curiosity. The key here is to provoke thoughtful reflection without judgment. It's a delicate balance of guidance and exploration that encourages clients to uncover truths about their existing beliefs and perceptions.

Alongside questioning, the integration of evidence-based facts is crucial. Encourage the examination of facts against cognitive distortions. For example, if a client believes "I am a failure," guide them to evaluate this belief by listing their achievements and contributions, however small they may appear. Merging fact with introspective questioning enables clients to shift from a perspective dominated by fear and trauma to one bolstered by insights and optimism.

Furthermore, engage clients in role-play exercises to explore new cognitive patterns. Role-play can provide an experiential learning environment where clients practice alternative reactions to negative thoughts or situations. Acting out scenarios grants clients the opportunity to rehearse new responses in a safe space, enhancing their ability to implement these changes outside of therapy. This method also taps into emotional learning, distinct from purely cognitive engagement, deepening the client's understanding and application of cognitive restructuring.

Visualization is another potent technique in cognitive restructuring. Guide clients in visualizing themselves handling distressing thoughts with newfound strategies. Visualization helps integrate cognitive shifts into their core identity, reinforcing the belief that they possess the skills to manage these thoughts effectively. It's a powerful tool in embedding these cognitive changes into the client's daily existence and routine.

As clients progress through cognitive restructuring, continual support and feedback from the therapist remain essential. Regularly revisiting thought records, reflections, and role-play enactments reinforces the learning process. The ongoing dialogue between client and therapist can help refine strategies, celebrate successes, and identify areas needing additional focus. Above all, building a strong therapeutic alliance fosters a collaborative journey of growth and healing.

Finally, it's crucial to understand that cognitive restructuring is not a one- size-fits-all solution. Tailor techniques to the unique needs of each client. Recognize that factors such as culture, personal history, and individual trauma experiences will influence the effectiveness of these techniques. Be mindful of the diverse backgrounds and take into consideration the personal nuances of each therapeutic relationship to maximize outcomes.

In sum, cognitive restructuring techniques serve as a framework within CPT for transforming destructive thought patterns into healthier cognitive processes. This transformation is not only vital for alleviating PTSD symptoms but also for empowering clients to reclaim control over their thoughts and lives. Through knowledgeable guidance and compassionate support, mental health professionals can facilitate this powerful journey toward healing and resilience, ultimately enabling clients to navigate their world with renewed clarity and strength.

Using Thought Records

In the journey of identifying and challenging maladaptive thoughts within Cognitive Processing Therapy (CPT), thought records serve as a critical, hands-on tool. They're not just worksheets to fill out; they offer a pathway to reframe the negative internal dialogues that perpetuate distress. Thought records help bridge the gap between experiencing automatic negative thoughts and developing healthier, more adaptive cognitive patterns. For clinicians working with clients who have PTSD, incorporating thought records into therapeutic practice can be a transformative process, both practically and emotionally.

Thought records facilitate this transformation by promoting awareness and understanding. They enable individuals to actively engage with their thought processes, moving from feelings of being out of control to a place of empowered insight. Practitioners find that when clients articulate their thoughts and corresponding emotions on paper, it opens a window into the cognitive processes that are otherwise left unexamined. The structure provided by a thought record guides clients to dissect intricate correlations between their thoughts, emotions, and behaviors, shedding light on patterns that might have persisted unrecognized.

Typically, a thought record includes several columns or sections where clients note the situation preceding the emotional response, the automatic thought that occurred, the emotions felt, and ultimately, the cognitive restructuring or more balanced thought. This structured approach can seem daunting at first, especially when dealing with the deeply ingrained habitual thinking patterns seen in trauma survivors. But with patient guidance and practice, clients learn that they're not merely reacting but actively reshaping their understanding of experiences.

When introducing thought records, it's helpful for therapists to model their use. Demonstrating how to translate a recent stressful situation into a thought record can ground an abstract idea into a tangible action. Clients benefit from seeing this firsthand, realizing that the exercise aims not for perfection but progress. A successful thought record session might explore self-identified themes such as "I am powerless" or "The world isn't safe," transitioning these perceptions toward more balanced alternatives like "I can exert control in many aspects of my life" or "There are elements of safety I can rely on."

Yet, therapists must approach the initial use with empathy, acknowledging any resistance or discomfort from clients. Trauma survivors might feel vulnerable because thought records require a degree of introspection that can initially be unsettling. Thus, it's crucial to create a non-judgmental, safe space where clients feel supported to explore their cognitive landscapes openly. Encouragement and affirmations are key components in fostering a trusting environment, encouraging clients to view mistakes or challenges as opportunities for growth, not failures.

Moreover, consistent integration of thought records into sessions can help develop them into a habit. Encouraging clients to work on these records between sessions makes the process less clinical and more a natural part of their daily routine. Gradually, they build cognitive resilience, equipping themselves to handle distressing thoughts more adeptly without always needing external intervention. Clinicians should consider intertwining this practice with technology, where digital thought records provide easy access and continuity of care, even beyond traditional session boundaries.

One of the most rewarding aspects for professionals is observing clients during therapy sessions when the revelations from their thought records come to light. Clients often express feelings of empowerment upon realizing the impact of their revised thoughts on their emotions and behaviors. This active engagement in reshaping their narrative can be profoundly liberating, reinforcing the therapeutic alliance and spurring further progress.

While the therapeutic impact of thought records is evident, therapists must remain mindful of their pacing. Overwhelming clients with too much introspection too quickly can be counterproductive. Instead, a gradual approach that tailors the complexity of the exercise to each client's readiness ensures that they aren't pushed beyond their emotional capacity. Incorporating feedback into session planning allows therapists to adjust and optimize how thought records are utilized throughout the therapy process.

Thought records are more than mere therapy tools; they are a gateway to self-discovery and healing. They're integral in the tapestry of cognitive restructuring techniques, providing a practical framework that enables those grappling with PTSD to challenge and change unhelpful cognitive patterns. For mental health professionals, mastery of guiding clients through the skillful use of thought records can significantly enhance therapeutic outcomes, paving the way for enduring behavioral and cognitive change. It's not just about what clients record on paper but what they learn to internalize, shaping a future that's not defined by past trauma but by a renewed and insightful perspective on self and the world.

CHAPTER
9

TEACHING EMOTIONAL PROCESSING

In the journey of cognitive processing therapy, teaching emotional processing stands as a crucial pillar, facilitating growth and healing for individuals grappling with trauma. This chapter delves into the nuanced understanding that emotions are not merely fleeting states to be endured but integral experiences to be observed, named, and understood.

By cultivating the ability to recognize and manage intense emotions, healthcare providers empower clients to build resilience and expand their emotional repertoire.

Teaching effective coping strategies nurtures a foundation upon which genuine emotional transformation can occur, allowing clients to engage with their experiences in a way that fosters healing and personal evolution. As therapists guide clients through this intricate terrain, they offer a compassionate scaffold, encouraging the development of skills needed to process emotions healthily and constructively. The empathetic lens through which this chapter is crafted aims to inspire mental health professionals to see the profound potential for change within each emotional discovery, reaffirming their vital role in nurturing a therapeutic space where emotional processing becomes both a journey and a beacon of hope.

Emotional Recognition

In the journey towards healing trauma, teaching emotional recognition stands as a pivotal step. Many individuals dealing with PTSD often grapple with an emotional landscape that feels hostile and perplexing. Understanding and acknowledging one's emotions can be daunting when the mind is ensnared by fear and distress triggered by past experiences. In this context, emotional recognition becomes a beacon of hope, guiding individuals toward self-awareness and recovery.

At its core, emotional recognition involves identifying and labeling emotions as they arise. This process might sound simple, but for someone who has endured trauma, it can feel akin to navigating a turbulent sea. Emotions intertwined with traumatic memories can blur into a chaotic whirlpool—an amalgamation of fear, anger, sadness, and confusion. Therefore, the first step in teaching this essential skill is creating a safe and supportive environment where individuals feel comfortable exploring their emotional state without judgment.

Health care providers and therapists can employ various strategies to facilitate emotional recognition. Encouraging patients to verbalize their feelings is a technique that underscores the importance of language in emotion. The act of naming an emotion—be it frustration, relief, or even numbness—provides cognitive clarity. Such clarity can help dismantle the overpowering nature of emotions, reducing them to manageable aspects of one's psyche that can be addressed rather than feared.

Another effective approach is implementing mindfulness practices. Through mindfulness, individuals learn to observe their emotions as transient states rather than permanent facets of their identity. This perspective fosters detachment from overwhelming emotions, allowing individuals to acknowledge their presence without becoming consumed by them. Techniques such as deep breathing, body scanning, or guided imagery can reinforce mindfulness, cultivating a non-judgmental awareness of the present moment.

In therapy sessions, visual aids like emotional charts or wheels can serve as practical tools for emotional recognition. These resources expand the emotional vocabulary beyond basic feelings of happiness, sadness, or anger and introduce nuances like anxiety, anticipation, or shame. By broadening the emotional lexicon, therapists empower individuals to pinpoint specific feelings more accurately, aiding in a deeper understanding and processing of their internal experiences. This specificity transforms abstract distress into defined entities that can be systematically addressed.

For some, emotional recognition might also involve decoding bodily sensations associated with different emotions. Trauma often manifests physically—tightness in the chest indicating anxiety, a knot in the stomach reflecting fear, or warmth radiating from the heart symbolizing joy. Teaching individuals to attune to these bodily signals can bridge the divide between their physical and emotional experiences. This holistic view of emotional recognition emphasizes the interconnectedness of mind and body, paving the way for a more unified therapeutic approach.

While these strategies lay the groundwork for emotional recognition, therapy is not a one-size-fits-all solution. Each individual's journey is unique, and adapting techniques to suit personal needs is paramount. Some might benefit from expressive arts therapy, where emotions are channeled through creative media like painting or music, while others might find solace in narrative forms, writing down emotional experiences to sift through them objectively.

It's important to acknowledge the role of cultural and social influences on emotional recognition. Different cultures may have distinct expressions and understandings of emotions, which can complicate the recognition process. Therapists must remain sensitive to these nuances, accommodating diverse emotional expressions and validating each individual's emotional experiences within their cultural context.

Encouraging patients to maintain a daily emotional journal is another constructive method. By recording their emotions consistently, individuals begin to notice patterns and triggers, which can prove invaluable in therapy. These insights can precipitate deeper discussions and explorations, enriching the therapeutic process and highlighting progress over time. The act of journaling itself often becomes a ritual of reflection, reinforcing the importance of emotional acknowledgment.

Ultimately, fostering emotional recognition is about more than just identifying feelings. It's about empowering individuals to reclaim control of their emotional narrative. In doing so, they move from being passive recipients of their emotions to active participants in shaping their emotional world. This empowerment is transformative—it offers a glimpse of stability amidst chaos and opens the door to healing.

As health care providers, researchers, and educators involved in this critical work, it's our privilege and responsibility to guide individuals through their emotional labyrinth. By prioritizing emotional recognition in therapy, we not only equip them with the tools to navigate their emotional landscape but also provide them with the foundation to cultivate resilience and well-being. Together, we contribute to a profound healing process that reverberates through the many facets of their lives.

Managing Intense Emotions

Emotional processing forms a cornerstone in reclaiming mental space, yet managing intense emotions can be one of the most taxing experiences for those dealing with PTSD. These emotions often seem overwhelming and, at times, destructive. For practitioners, helping patients navigate these feelings isn't just about teaching them to weather the storm; it's about empowering them to understand their emotional landscape and the physical sensations that accompany it. This chapter aims to arm healthcare providers, researchers, and mental health professionals with strategies to support patients effectively, fostering both resilience and clarity in the face of emotional upheaval.

A critical step in managing intense emotions is the recognition and validation of those feelings. Patients commonly experience emotions like anger, sadness, fear, and guilt, often intensified by traumatic experiences. Saying to them, "You're not alone in feeling this way" can be a crucial first step. Validating their emotions not only strengthens the therapeutic alliance, a key focus in earlier chapters, but also establishes a foundation on which patients can begin exploring their emotions further.

Once emotions are acknowledged, the next focus is understanding and dissecting these emotions without being consumed by them. For therapists, guiding the patient through this exploration involves helping them find the language to articulate complex and often conflicting feelings. Patients might not initially differentiate between feeling anxious and unsafe, or sad and ashamed. Helping them refine their emotional vocabulary allows them to better pinpoint what they're truly experiencing. Often, journaling or expressive writing can be utilized as a tool here, allowing patients the space to reflect upon and organize their emotions.

Behavioral techniques also play a significant role in managing emotions. When heightened emotions latch onto thought patterns, cognitive restructuring, a technique introduced earlier, aids patients in reframing these thoughts. By focusing on cognitive distortions that magnify intense emotions, therapists can help patients recognize and challenge spirals of negative thinking. For those dealing with anger, this might mean uncovering underlying hurt or frustration that has festered unacknowledged.

Self-regulation is another skill crucial to managing intense emotions. Breathing exercises, progressive muscle relaxation, and mindfulness can reduce the physiological symptoms that typically accompany heightened emotions. These techniques empower patients by providing immediate, tangible ways to regulate their bodies' responses, thus indirectly calming the mind. For many patients, incorporating regular mindfulness practices into their daily routine not only helps manage acute emotional distress but also enhances overall well-being.

However, while these techniques provide tools for individual management of emotions, the relational aspect of emotional processing cannot be overlooked. Therapy provides the safe space necessary for patients to engage in controlled exposure to emotions within the context of interpersonal relationships. Role-playing scenarios and therapist modeling are strategies that can help patients learn to express emotions constructively in real-world interactions. It's important for professionals to remember that growth often occurs in the context of relationships, and thus encouraging patients to seek and cultivate supportive relationships outside of therapy is invaluable.

It is essential for mental health professionals to understand that managing intense emotions isn't about suppression but about integration. Patients should be encouraged to view emotions as informative and integral components of their identity rather than adversaries to be subdued. This shift in perspective can lead to profound therapeutic breakthroughs, fostering a sense of empowerment rather than victimhood. Additionally, techniques borrowed from acceptance and commitment therapy can be used to support this understanding, helping individuals hold their emotions with compassion while continuing to pursue meaningful life goals.

Lastly, healthcare providers must acknowledge and manage their emotional responses during sessions. The multifaceted nature of intense emotions in clients can evoke strong countertransference reactions. Therapists must be vigilant in recognizing their emotional responses and employ strategies such as supervision and peer support to ensure they remain effective and unimpeded in their work. Creating a reflective practice of one's responses aids in maintaining the therapeutic alliance and modeling emotional management skills for patients.

Successful management of intense emotions in PTSD treatment is a dynamic process that intertwines emotional literacy, cognitive restructuring, physiological regulation, and interpersonal relationships. By integrating these strategies, therapists can assist patients in not only navigating their emotional experiences but also harnessing them as a source of strength and insight. The goal is to equip patients with the capacity to embrace their full emotional spectrum, thus restoring a sense of control and paving the way for mental and emotional freedom.

Coping Strategies

In the realm of teaching emotional processing, coping strategies hold a pivotal role. They are not merely survival mechanisms but are better understood as tools for thriving amidst adversity. For those working through the tumult of PTSD, learning effective ways to cope is essential. It's about transforming overwhelming experiences into manageable parts and encouraging empowerment in the face of trauma.

Coping strategies can be the cornerstone of emotional resilience. These strategies help bridge the gap between recognizing emotions and taking constructive action. As health care providers and mental health professionals, it's crucial to equip patients with a variety of coping mechanisms to navigate the complexities of their internal world. This approach empowers individuals to move through distress with a sense of control, rather than feeling controlled by it.

A fundamental component of teaching coping strategies involves helping individuals identify and understand their emotions. Before one can manage their emotional responses, they need to recognize and validate them. This self-awareness serves as the first step in developing effective coping responses. Encouraging patients to label their emotions accurately is essential in this process. It provides clarity in chaos, turning nebulous feelings into tangible experiences that can be addressed more readily.

Once emotions are recognized, the focus shifts to coping strategies that can be employed in real-time. One key technique is grounding exercises. Grounding techniques can anchor an individual in the present moment, providing tangible connections to reality. Techniques such as deep breathing, focusing on sensory experiences, or employing mindfulness can disrupt the cycle of negative thoughts and bring attention back to the present.

In addition to grounding, developing a patient's emotional resilience will often include encouraging the use of cognitive reframing. This involves identifying negative thought patterns and reshaping them into more positive or realistic perspectives. By challenging distorted cognitions, individuals can alleviate emotional distress, reducing the intensity of their emotional responses and ultimately altering behavior patterns.

Support systems, both personal and communal, are indispensable in this journey. Fostering connections with supportive others can offer validation and encouragement, often serving as a lifeline during trying times. It is important for health care providers to guide individuals in building and utilizing their support networks effectively. Engaging with family, friends, or support groups can enhance an individual's ability to cope by providing differing perspectives and shared experiences.

Moreover, the utilization of creative outlets can serve as an effective coping mechanism. Encouraging individuals to explore activities like art, music, or writing can provide an alternative means of expression. These methods often enable the expression of thoughts and emotions that might be difficult to articulate otherwise. Creative outlets can be therapeutic, offering an opportunity for reflection and personal insight.

Cultivating self-compassion is another critical aspect of teaching coping strategies. Encouraging individuals to treat themselves with kindness amidst suffering can counteract self-critical tendencies. Self-compassion fosters a more forgiving and nurturing internal environment, promoting healing as individuals learn to accept their human imperfections.

Physical activity is a coping strategy that cannot be overlooked. Regular exercise has been demonstrated to have beneficial effects on mood and stress levels. As part of a comprehensive approach to emotional processing, incorporating physical exercise can aid in managing symptoms of anxiety and depression commonly associated with PTSD. Simple activities like walking or stretching can make a significant difference in a person's emotional well-being.

Yet, not every strategy works for every individual, and that's where personalization is key. Tailoring coping mechanisms to fit the unique needs and preferences of each person is essential for their success. Encouraging patients to explore various strategies until they find what resonates is part of this personalized approach.

The role of technology also comes into play. Digital tools and apps designed for mental health can provide easy access to coping strategies. These resources can be beneficial in reinforcing skills learned in therapy, offering guided exercises, and tracking progress. Technology, when harnessed appropriately, can enhance the accessibility and applicability of coping strategies for individuals working through PTSD.

Ultimately, teaching coping strategies involves guiding individuals toward proactive, rather than reactive, responses to emotional challenges. By building a repertoire of effective coping mechanisms, individuals are better equipped to face their triggers and manage their emotional states constructively. The journey of emotional processing becomes one of empowerment, turning what was once perceived as insurmountable into manageable steps toward healing and growth.

As educators and clinicians, our task is to foster a supportive environment where these coping strategies can be explored and integrated into the daily lives of those we serve. It's about instilling hope and demonstrating that, despite past trauma, a future filled with resilience and emotional stability is achievable.

CHAPTER 10

TRAUMA NARRATIVES

Creating trauma narratives is a powerful and transformative process in Cognitive Processing Therapy (CPT). This chapter delves into the significance of guiding patients through the often daunting but healing journey of articulating their trauma account. At its core, constructing a trauma narrative involves the detailed writing or recounting of the traumatic events that someone has experienced.

This exercise isn't merely about revisiting painful memories; it's about gaining agency and allowing fragmented experiences to coalesce into a coherent story. As patients narrate their experiences, they begin to process emotions and confront avoidance—a natural yet counterproductive response to trauma. The role of the therapist here is pivotal, facilitating an environment of empathy and safety while encouraging exploration of the patient's internal landscape.

Through reading and processing the narratives, patients can challenge maladaptive beliefs and break free from the constraints trauma has imposed, gradually reclaiming their mental autonomy and creating space for recovery. This method not only fosters insight but also serves as a crucial stepping stone toward empowerment and healing, equipping mental health professionals with the tools to support their patients effectively.

Mriting the Trauma Account

The journey of writing the trauma account is both delicate and powerful, acting as a bridge between acknowledging past experiences and facilitating deep healing. For health care providers, educators, and mental health professionals, guiding individuals through this process demands a nuanced understanding of the personal and psychological barriers that may arise. While the task at hand seems straightforward—write the story of the trauma—it involves navigating a landscape interwoven with avoidance, fear, and pain.

In crafting a trauma account, the first and perhaps most significant step is creating a therapeutic environment where patients feel safe enough to revisit their stories. This is crucial since safety fosters the courage needed to confront vulnerabilities. It's essential to communicate empathy and understanding, validating the patient's emotions and experiences. Such an environment encourages openness and support, forming the groundwork for a sincere narrative.

Importantly, the trauma account is not written all at once. Patients often begin with fragmented memories, scattered like pieces of a puzzle. Encouraging them to start with whatever memory feels most accessible helps break the initial resistance. This might involve recalling a specific detail, a feeling, or a sensory experience. Gradually expanding these fragments into a fuller narrative, while avoiding the pressure to adhere to a chronological order, can alleviate the daunting nature of the task.

Professionals should emphasize that there is no right or wrong way to tell a trauma story. Writing can progress at the patient's pace, honoring their personal limits and boundaries. The content and flow should mirror their comfort level and readiness. It's vital to remind them that revisiting trauma doesn't mean reliving it. The goal is to foster a new relationship with the past, one where they have control over the narrative.

An effective strategy to support individuals through this endeavor is the use of structured writing prompts or guided questions, which can facilitate deeper engagement with the narrative. These prompts, however, should be adaptable, flexible to the unique contexts and emotional landscapes of each patient. Guiding questions such as, "What was the most challenging part of the experience?" or "How did you cope in that moment?" can provide direction without overwhelming the patient.

Throughout this process, it is essential to be attuned to signs of distress or re-traumatization. Therapists must monitor the emotional and physiological responses of their patients, ready to intervene with grounding techniques and coping strategies if necessary. The goal is to maintain a balance between emotional exposure and containment, ensuring that writing the trauma account remains a therapeutic, rather than harmful, endeavor.

Moreover, reading the written account aloud in therapy sessions can offer additional therapeutic benefits, helping patients process emotions verbally and gain insight into their experiences. This also provides an opportunity for therapists to offer immediate support and feedback, facilitate reflection, and address any emerging themes or patterns in the narrative. However, it's important to proceed with sensitivity, giving patients the choice to share what they've written or hold it privately.

For mental health professionals, fostering a sense of empowerment is crucial. Patients should be assured that they are the architects of their own stories. Encouraging them to identify parts of their narrative where they demonstrated resilience or resourcefulness can help shift focus from victimhood to survivorship. This reframing can enhance self-esteem and rekindle a sense of agency and control—the cornerstones of psychological healing.

In writing and revising the trauma account, patients often discover new layers of understanding and meaning. They may find connections between past experiences and current behavioral patterns, attitudes, or beliefs. Such insights can be pivotal in cognitive restructuring, allowing for the reformation of healthier thought processes and the release of distorted cognitions, which are addressed later in therapy.

The role of the therapist in this process is multi-faceted: a supportive guide, an empathetic listener, and sometimes a co-explorer of meanings. Establishing a collaborative dynamic can strengthen therapeutic alliance, fostering a partnership built on trust and mutual goals. As narratives evolve, therapists may assist in identifying and challenging maladaptive beliefs, enriching the therapeutic journey.

Writing the trauma account ultimately serves as a foundation for subsequent therapeutic work. It sets the stage for delving deeper into emotional processing and challenging maladaptive beliefs, reinforcing the notion that the trauma does not define the individual. It is a potent exercise in self-exploration, self-compassion, and eventually, self- liberation.

As you facilitate this transformative process, remember the profound significance of empathy and patience. Each narrative, while a recount of adversity and suffering, also embodies the journey towards recovery and renewal. By encouraging and supporting the writing of the trauma account, therapists and mental health professionals empower individuals to reclaim their stories, their identities, and ultimately, their lives.

Reading and Processing

Reading and processing a trauma narrative is a foundational task in Cognitive Processing Therapy

(CPT), serving as both an instrument of healing and a compass guiding therapeutic direction. It's a delicate art and science, combining empathetic listening with cognitive restructuring to help individuals reclaim their narratives without the persistent shadow of trauma. This process begins with creating a safe space, both physically and emotionally, where individuals feel seen and heard without judgment. It is within this refuge that they bravely revisit and confront their stories.

The process of reading the trauma narrative begins with acknowledging the dual role of memory and emotion. Memories fragment under the assault of trauma, and the narrative, as expressed, might first appear disjointed or unclear. Each word or pause may carry layers of meaning, from palpable fear to repressed anger. The therapist's role is to help the individual piece together their story like a puzzle, guiding them to recognize not only the factual aspects of the trauma but also the emotional imprints left behind. This is not merely an intellectual exercise; it involves the holistic integration of thoughts and feelings.

Empathy is the bridge that connects the therapist to the trauma survivor during this reading process. As the narrative unfolds, it can trigger intense emotions for both parties; therefore, maintaining composure while providing support is crucial. Practitioners must balance empathy with professional boundaries to create a therapeutic alliance that empowers the individual to reflect on their experiences constructively. Active listening and validation are key, as they encourage trust and openness necessary for therapeutic progress.

One of the challenging aspects of processing lies in identifying cognitive distortions within the narrative. Trauma tends to warp perception, often anchoring individuals in loops of guilt, shame, or blame. These distorted thoughts influence how the narrative is told and understood. A significant part of therapeutic work involves gently challenging these distortions, helping individuals widen their perspective and find new, healthier ways to interpret their experiences.

This phase of therapy is not about erasing memories but about reframing and integrating them. The narrative's power lies in how it's told and understood—transforming from a source of distress into an empowering account of survival and growth. Processing this narrative helps individuals establish a coherent sense of self and a renewed understanding of their world, allowing for healing that embraces the totality of their experience.

Therapists often witness breathtaking moments of revelation and resilience during this process. As trauma is painstakingly woven into the broader tapestry of a person's life story, it's essential to recognize and honor the courage it takes to confront such personal history. Each session, each narrative reading, is a testament to human strength and the transformative power of therapy.

Of course, not every session will be smooth, and the emotional labor required from both client and therapist can be substantial. However, by respecting the pace that each individual is comfortable with, practitioners can help them navigate through resistance and avoidance. These hurdles are not failures but necessary parts of the healing process that signify engagement with deeply-rooted issues.

Moreover, therapists must remain observant and flexible, open to the ebb and flow of emotional expression that accompanies narrative processing. By adopting a stance of curiosity rather than prescriptive direction, therapists can facilitate discovery and insight without imposing their interpretations. This approach nurtures autonomy, encouraging individuals to reclaim their narratives authentically.

Engaging in this work requires constant reflection and learning on the therapist's part too. They benefit from supervision and peer support to process their emotional responses and sustain their well-being.

Indeed, the act of bearing witness to another 's trauma narrative can be transformative for the therapist as well, bearing the dual obligation of facilitating healing and maintaining self-care.

Ultimately, reading and processing trauma narratives is about fostering resilience — both in the faces of those we work with and within ourselves. It is a journey marked by mutual discovery, where recounting pain becomes an act of defiance and hope. It's an invitation to transcend past suffering and embrace the possibility of a future defined not by trauma, but by resilience and renewal, helping individuals reclaim the narratives they were destined to live.

Addressing Avoidance

In the delicate process of creating trauma narratives, avoidance often stands as a formidable barrier. It manifests in various forms, from subtle distraction techniques to outright refusal to engage with distressing memories. Addressing avoidance is not merely about confronting these narratives directly; it's about gently guiding individuals to a place where they can safely explore their experiences without judgment or excessive distress.

Understanding avoidance begins with recognizing it as a natural, albeit often maladaptive, response to trauma. People who've experienced trauma may instinctively evade reminders of their painful experiences because facing them can feel overwhelming. It's not uncommon for individuals to adopt conscious or unconscious strategies to steer clear of thoughts, feelings, or situations associated with their trauma. This adaptive mechanism is the mind's way of protecting itself from the potential inundation of overwhelming emotions. However, while this may offer temporary relief, it can perpetuate the cycle of avoidance, ultimately exacerbating symptoms over time.

Clinicians must validate these avoidance strategies as protective measures that once served a purpose, albeit one that no longer facilitates healing. An empathetic stance helps foster a therapeutic alliance, allowing the individual to feel safe and understood. From this foundation, the process of addressing avoidance can begin in earnest.

One effective method involves incremental exposure. This controlled exposure isn't about throwing individuals into the deep end but rather about facilitating gentle, manageable engagements with their trauma narratives. This might start with cognitive exercises that address avoidance on a more abstract level, gradually edged closer to direct engagement. For instance, a patient might initially describe unrelated minor stressors, building confidence simply in recounting difficult situations.

As patients become more comfortable, the exposure can begin to incorporate elements of their trauma narrative itself. It's crucial this is done at a pace that respects the individual's readiness, as pushing too quickly can reinforce avoidance and destabilize the therapeutic process. Encouraging autonomy in dictating this pace empowers patients, granting them a sense of control that's often erased by trauma.

Practitioners must also be particularly adept at recognizing avoidance when it masquerades as something else. Sometimes, seemingly cooperative behaviors may hide avoidance. A patient over-intellectualizing their trauma or continuously focusing on unrelated tangential issues might be avoiding deeper engagement. Here, the clinician's skill in gently steering conversations back without causing defensiveness is paramount.

Another approach involves the incorporation of motivational interviewing techniques. This strategy is crucial for creating awareness and understanding of avoidance's impact on recovery and how facing discomfort can eventually lead to relief. By emphasizing the patient's intrinsic motivations and goals, clinicians can help them find personal reasons to overcome avoidance, making the arduous process of recall and processing more purposeful and less daunting.

Moreover, addressing avoidance requires a holistic understanding of each person's unique coping mechanisms. Cultural backgrounds, personal history, and individual personalities play significant roles in shaping how one might manifest avoidance. For instance, certain cultural contexts might stigmatize emotional expression, inadvertently fostering avoidance. In such cases, culturally sensitive adaptations in technique can make a profound difference in engagement.

The use of thought records and other cognitive processing tools can be instrumental in this regard. These tools direct patients to dissect their avoidance behaviors in a structured manner, exploring not only the act of avoidance itself but the underlying beliefs and fears driving these actions. As patients regularly practice noting and challenging instances of avoidance, they develop a clearer awareness of their patterns, equipping them with the means to disrupt these patterns more effectively.

It's equally important to address the physiological components of avoidance. Stress response systems in the body, activated during traumatic incidents, can make cognitive processing of trauma narratives difficult. Techniques such as mindfulness and relaxation can assist in modulating these physiological responses, providing a more conducive environment for processing trauma narratives.

The path through avoidance is often non-linear, fraught with setbacks. These moments should be seen less as failures and more as opportunities for recalibration. A compassionate and patient approach emphasizes these points, reinforcing that healing is inherently a process, and a non-linear one at that.

Importantly, collaboration with the patient in establishing a clear framework for sessions can reduce the fear of the unknown, which often bolsters avoidance. Shared goals, transparency in methods, and patient involvement in planning each session lend themselves to a predictable and safe therapeutic environment.

Finally, regular reflection on progress, no matter how small, is vital in sustaining motivation. Highlighting achievements in facing avoidance and processing trauma narratives can build resilience and a positive outlook on recovery. As patients see the tangible rewards of their efforts— improved functioning, diminished PTSD symptoms, enhanced quality of life— they are more likely to break free from the chains of avoidance.

Addressing avoidance in trauma narratives is less about forcing confrontation and more about inviting engagement. It requires a blend of patience, strategy, empathy, and skill from clinicians. With these elements in place, patients can gradually reclaim agency over their narratives, confront avoidance with confidence, and ultimately, move towards a place of healing and recovery.

CHAPTER 11

ADDRESSING MALADAPTIVE BELIEFS

As we journey into addressing maladaptive beliefs in the realm of Cognitive Processing Therapy (CPT), it's essential to recognize the power these beliefs hold over an individual's experience of trauma. These deep-rooted convictions often distort a person's view of themselves, others, and the world, fueling feelings of hopelessness and perpetuating the cycle of distress. Our goal as mental health professionals is to help patients identify these core beliefs, bringing them to light where they can be challenged and transformed. By encouraging clients to question the validity of their distorted cognitions, we open up possibilities for healing and growth. The process involves empathically guiding individuals to reinforce positive beliefs, ones that empower rather than imprison. This chapter provides strategies for facilitating these crucial cognitive shifts, anchoring them in a foundation of trust and collaboration, paving the way for lasting change and a reclaimed sense of agency.

In Cognitive Processing Therapy (CPT), the process of identifying and addressing maladaptive beliefs is not a quick fix, but rather a gradual and deeply transformative journey. Research indicates that trauma not only affects emotional well-being, but can also lead to significant cognitive changes that influence how individuals perceive and interpret the world. These shifts in thought patterns often serve to reinforce feelings of helplessness or guilt, as trauma survivors come to believe that the traumatic event was a reflection of their own inadequacies. The therapeutic approach, therefore, focuses not only on alleviating the immediate symptoms of trauma but also on disrupting the maladaptive cognitive patterns that contribute to long-term suffering. The goal is to provide patients with the cognitive tools necessary to challenge these self-limiting beliefs and reframe their understanding of their trauma and self-worth.

A fascinating aspect of the CPT process is how it draws on both cognitive-behavioral principles and trauma-informed care to achieve lasting change. ognitive restructuring, a core component of CPT, involves helping clients identify cognitive distortions such as overgeneralization, catastrophizing, and black-and-white thinking. These distortions can trap individuals in a cycle of negative thought patterns, preventing them from moving forward. By encouraging clients to scrutinize these thoughts and evaluate the evidence supporting them, CPT helps them recognize the inaccuracies in their beliefs. This approach not only fosters healthier cognitive patterns but also encourages a shift from a passive stance toward one of active self-reflection and empowerment.

Furthermore, CPT's emphasis on collaboration between therapist and client is essential for the healing process. Research consistently shows that the therapeutic alliance—the relationship between therapist and patient—plays a pivotal role in treatment success. By creating an environment of trust and mutual respect, therapists provide a safe space for clients to explore their most vulnerable thoughts and feelings. This collaborative approach also reinforces the idea that healing is a shared process, with both the therapist and client working together to challenge and modify distorted beliefs. This partnership enhances clients' sense of agency, which is crucial for fostering a sense of control and empowerment in their healing journey.

As individuals begin to internalize healthier, more adaptive beliefs, they may notice a profound shift not only in their thoughts but also in their emotions and behaviors. Research in neuroplasticity suggests that the brain has an incredible ability to reorganize itself in response to new learning and experiences. This means that, as clients challenge their maladaptive beliefs and replace them with more realistic and positive thoughts, they are literally rewiring their brain. Over time, these cognitive shifts lead to changes in emotional regulation and coping strategies, helping individuals build resilience in the face of future stressors. By guiding clients to challenge deeply ingrained negative beliefs, CPT provides not just relief from trauma, but also the tools for creating a healthier, more balanced future.

Identifying Core Beliefs

Identifying core beliefs is pivotal in addressing the intricate web of maladaptive thinking that often accompanies trauma. Core beliefs are the deeply held perceptions individuals have about themselves, others, and the world. They form the lens through which experiences are interpreted and are rooted in early life, shaped by our interactions and environments.

When trauma occurs, these beliefs can become maladaptive, leading to distorted thinking patterns that negatively impact mental health and well- being. Recognizing these foundational thoughts is crucial for meaningful therapeutic progress, as it helps unravel the negative narratives that perpetuate distress and dysfunction.

Core beliefs are not immediately evident; they lie beneath the surface of conscious thought and require careful exploration. They often manifest in automatic thoughts and emotional responses to everyday situations, acting as an internal script that guides behavior. For instance, a person with a belief of being unworthy may interpret neutral interactions as rejecting, reinforcing feelings of inadequacy. Identifying these deep-seated convictions involves peeling back layers of cognition to uncover the underlying assumptions that govern how individuals perceive themselves in relation to their world. This process can be both enlightening and challenging, as it requires a willingness to confront long-standing narratives.

Therapists play a crucial role in facilitating this exploration by creating a compassionate and nonjudgmental environment. Through guided questioning and reflective dialogue, therapists encourage clients to articulate their automatic thoughts and examine the evidence supporting these beliefs. Techniques such as Socratic questioning help clients to scrutinize the validity of their assumptions and consider alternative perspectives. For example, a therapist might ask, "What evidence do you have to support this belief?" or "How might someone else view this situation differently?" Such inquiries challenge clients to rethink their narratives, opening the door to cognitive restructuring and belief modification.

One of the initial steps in identifying core beliefs involves recognizing patterns in thoughts and behaviors. Clients are encouraged to keep thought records, a tool that captures situations, emotions, and automatic thoughts in real-time. By analyzing these records, clients and therapists can pinpoint recurring themes and begin to trace them back to the underlying core beliefs. This process often reveals common cognitive distortions, such as overgeneralization or catastrophic thinking, that can be traced back to these core convictions. Bringing these beliefs to consciousness allows clients to critically evaluate their validity and impact, paving the way for cognitive shifts.

The process of identifying core beliefs is not linear; it often involves revisiting and reformulating understandings as therapy progresses. As clients gain insights and experience shifts in perspective, they may uncover additional layers of beliefs that require examination. This dynamic process underscores the importance of sustained and flexible therapeutic engagement, adapting to the evolving needs of the client. It's essential that therapists remain attuned to these shifts, validating the client's journey and providing support as they navigate through complex cognitive terrain.

It's important to acknowledge that core beliefs aren't inherently negative. They serve vital functions, helping individuals make sense of their experiences. However, when molded by trauma, they can become overly rigid or distorted, contributing to ongoing psychological distress. By identifying and addressing these beliefs, therapists empower clients to reconstruct their cognitive frameworks in more adaptive and flexible ways. This restructuring fosters resilience, enabling clients to approach life with a renewed sense of agency and possibility.

Adapting therapeutic approaches to the unique context of each client is vital in uncovering core beliefs. Cultural, social, and personal dimensions influence how beliefs form and manifest. Therapists should remain sensitive to these factors, integrating culturally-informed practices that honor the client's lived experiences. Engaging in culturally sensitive dialogue can illuminate diverse belief systems, allowing for a more comprehensive understanding of the client's internal world. Such sensitivity not only enriches the therapeutic process but also affirms the client's identity and experience.

A critical component of identifying core beliefs involves exploring the emotional responses they provoke. Emotions often serve as indicators of underlying beliefs, offering clues to their nature and origin. Therapists can guide clients in connecting their emotional experiences to specific thoughts and beliefs, helping demystify the emotional landscape. By understanding the emotional triggers linked to core beliefs, clients gain greater awareness of how these beliefs influence their lives. This awareness is a catalyst for change, fostering emotional regulation and adaptive emotional processing.

As therapists work with clients to identify and transform core beliefs, they foster a sense of empowerment and competency. Clients who recognize their ability to challenge and revise these beliefs often experience a renewed sense of self-efficacy and hope. The act of examining and reshaping core beliefs not only alleviates distress but can also engender significant personal growth. Clients learn that while they cannot change the past, they have the power to redefine how they understand and interact with the world.

In helping clients identify their core beliefs, therapists also model a way of engaging with the world that is curious, compassionate, and open- minded. They demonstrate that beliefs are susceptible to change, encouraging clients to adopt a more flexible and dynamic approach to thinking. While identifying core beliefs may initially bring discomfort, it ultimately leads to a more nuanced and liberated view of oneself and one's potential. As clients embark on this journey, they move towards a more integrated and authentic sense of self, capable of facing life's challenges with strength and resilience.

By addressing core beliefs, therapists and clients embark on a partnership aimed at transforming pain into possibility. The process of identifying these beliefs is more than an intellectual exercise; it's a profound exploration of the self that can bring about healing at the deepest levels. Through this work, clients learn to confront and rewrite the narratives that have defined them, stepping into a future not bound by past traumas but inspired by newfound understanding and strength. This transformation marks a fundamental step in reclaiming mental space and time, advancing toward a more fulfilling and empowered life.

As clients begin to recognize the fluidity of their beliefs, they start to see that the way they view themselves, others, and the world is not fixed but can evolve over time. This awareness fosters a sense of hope, as clients realize they have the power to reshape their cognitive frameworks and ultimately their life experiences. By encouraging a mindset of curiosity, therapists invite clients to explore different perspectives and engage with their thoughts in a more open and less judgmental way. This process aligns with the concept of neuroplasticity, which suggests that the brain's connections can be rewired with consistent practice. Just as muscles grow stronger with exercise, cognitive flexibility strengthens with ongoing practice, allowing individuals to respond to challenges with greater adaptability and emotional balance.

The partnership between therapist and client in this work not only helps dismantle maladaptive beliefs but also provides an opportunity for the creation of new, empowering narratives. This shift in perspective allows clients to move beyond the confines of their past trauma and start envisioning a future rooted in personal growth and self-compassion. Research on trauma recovery emphasizes the importance of finding meaning in the aftermath of traumatic events, and by reinterpreting old beliefs, clients can craft stories of survival, strength, and resilience. This process of self-reconstruction allows them to redefine their identity in a way that acknowledges the pain they've experienced while also celebrating their capacity for healing and transformation. Through this journey, individuals are no longer defined by their trauma but are empowered to thrive beyond it.

Challenging Distorted Cognitions

In the journey of addressing maladaptive beliefs, one of the most pivotal tasks is challenging distorted cognitions. These cognitions often serve as the internal narratives that perpetuate distress in individuals who have experienced trauma. As mental health professionals, our role is to work with clients to unearth and question these deeply rooted thought patterns. This process can significantly alter the client's perceptions and emotional responses, ultimately mitigating the overwhelming power of trauma.

Understanding how these thoughts manifest and affect behavior is key to guiding clients toward healing.

Distorted cognitions typically arise as a result of the misinterpretation of traumatic events. Clients often generalize or overemphasize negative aspects while dismissing or minimizing positive experiences. For instance, a survivor might believe they are wholly responsible for the traumatic event, ignoring contextual factors beyond their control. Such cognitive distortions can appear as all-or-nothing thinking, catastrophizing, or personalization, among others. Our objective is to help clients identify these faulty patterns and understand their impact on mental well-being.

A practical approach to challenging distorted cognitions starts with education. Explain to clients how their cognitive processes interpret events and how these interpretations can become skewed. You might discuss how the brain's natural reaction to trauma can lead to irrational and negative thought patterns. By understanding the science behind these responses, clients can feel empowered, rather than defective.

Once clients recognize their cognitive distortions, the next step is to work collaboratively to question and reframe these thoughts. Encourage them to examine evidence for and against these beliefs critically. It's essential to foster an environment where clients feel safe to voice their concerns without judgment. Providing examples and sharing relatable stories can facilitate this exploration. Highlighting times when their assumptions were proven incorrect can also encourage a shift in perspective.

Consider employing thought records as a tool to document and dismantle distorted cognitions. These records serve as a roadmap for individuals to track their thoughts, emotions, and behaviors in response to specific situations. Over time, these entries can reveal patterns and areas for focused intervention. Encourage clients to ask questions such as, "Is there an alternative explanation?" or "What would I say to a friend in this situation?" These prompts help cultivate a more balanced and realistic outlook.

It is crucial to recognize that challenging distorted cognitions requires persistence and patience. Change doesn't happen overnight, and clients may resist initially. However, by continuously applying these techniques and remaining supportive, clients can develop healthier thinking patterns. This transformation aids in reducing symptoms of PTSD and enhances overall functionality.

Integration of empirical evidence can bolster the reframing process. Discuss studies or findings from cognitive-behavioral research that support the effectiveness of examining and altering thought patterns. Knowing that others have successfully navigated similar challenges can inspire hope and reinforce the desire for change. Reinforcing positive beliefs, once distorted cognitions have been challenged, helps in consolidating the newfound clarity.

Moreover, offering alternative frameworks, like replacing self-blame with self-compassion, can further aid in reshaping clients' thought processes. By shifting from a place of judgment to a stance of understanding, clients can learn to forgive themselves and embrace a more nurturing self-view. This process not only involves cognitive shifts but often requires emotional reconciliation with past events.

The therapist's role in this journey cannot be overstated. By modeling empathy, offering validation, and providing a safe space, therapists can effectively guide clients through this transformative process. Building a strong therapeutic alliance is fundamental in ensuring clients feel supported as they confront and revise their distorted cognitions.

In conclusion, challenging distorted cognitions is a cornerstone of addressing maladaptive beliefs. As health care providers and mental health professionals, we are uniquely positioned to guide clients through this process. By combining psychoeducation with practical tools like thought records, fostering a supportive environment, and emphasizing self-compassion, we can empower clients to reclaim their mental space and lead more fulfilling lives. Overcoming these cognitive hurdles is an essential step toward healing and realizing personal growth.

Reinforcing Positive Beliefs

In the aftermath of trauma, the landscapes of the mind often shift toward shadows, where negative beliefs about oneself, the world, and the future can take root. Yet, amidst these shadows, therapy offers a pathway back into the light, with reinforcing positive beliefs playing a pivotal role in recovery. This transformative process is not just about challenging the negative; it's about cultivating, nurturing, and solidifying the positive. It invites individuals to rediscover hope, reframe their perceptions, and ultimately reclaim their sense of agency and worth.

Understanding the nature of positive beliefs is the cornerstone of their reinforcement. Positive beliefs are not mere affirmations or empty platitudes; they are deeply held convictions that can serve as buffers against distressing emotions and maladaptive thought patterns. They can encompass a broad spectrum, from beliefs about personal competence and self-worth to those about safety and trust in others. As therapists, our task is to guide individuals in identifying these beliefs amidst the rubble of trauma and supporting them in anchoring these beliefs firmly in their psyche.

Therapists play an active role in the empowerment process, facilitating the discovery and reinforcement of positive beliefs. We start by creating a nurturing environment where patients feel safe to explore areas of potential strength and resilience. In these spaces, self-exploration can lead to revelations. For example, a patient with PTSD may begin to recognize their inherent resilience by recounting instances where they acted courageously in the face of adversity. By doing so, they may begin to establish a foundation upon which positive beliefs can be built.

Active dialogue forms a crucial part of reinforcing positive beliefs. Through collaborative discussions, therapists and patients work together to identify, challenge, and reformulate distorted cognitions that have held sway for too long. During these exchanges, instances of personal success and overcoming are highlighted, and positive feedback is provided, reinforcing the idea that change is not only possible but already happening in incremental ways.

Incorporating experiential exercises can further solidify these positive beliefs. Role-playing scenarios, mindfulness exercises, and visualization techniques are powerful tools in this regard. They encourage individuals to experience potential positive outcomes, bridging the gap between belief and reality. Such exercises not only reinforce cognitive shift but also build emotional resilience, guiding patients to feel the changes they're striving toward.

Positive beliefs also thrive on the narrative voice. What stories do patients tell themselves? The process of rewriting their trauma narratives to include elements of strength, perseverance, and survival can be immensely empowering. This narrative reframing allows individuals to interlace positive beliefs with their experiences, transforming their overall self-concept and worldview.

Families and communities also play a significant role in this process. As therapists, bringing these entities into the therapeutic fold can amplify positive reinforcement. Family sessions or community support groups can provide external validation of developing positive beliefs, as loved ones and peers reflect back strengths and areas of growth. Here, positive beliefs are not just self-generated; they are mirrored and reinforced within a larger relational context.

Consistency is key in this journey. The repeated practice of identifying and reinforcing positive beliefs helps solidify these thought patterns, turning them from transient hopes into steadfast beliefs. Regularly revisiting these beliefs during therapy sessions ensures they are being maintained and, when necessary, adapted to new challenges or insights.

This reinforcement process requires patience and persistence—from therapists and patients alike. Challenges, setbacks, and moments of doubt are natural; they are not indicative of failure. Instead, they provide opportunities to deepen the work, refocusing on the positive beliefs that have already taken root, and nurturing them further.

It's critical that therapists maintain an empathetic and non-judgmental stance throughout this process. Understanding the weight of the past traumas and the subsequent struggle to cultivate positivity requires sensitivity and compassion. By modeling these qualities, therapists create a space where patients feel understood rather than judged, and encouraged rather than pressured.

Ultimately, as patients begin to own their positive beliefs, a remarkable transformation takes place. They move from merely surviving in the aftermath of trauma to actively crafting a life with renewed purpose and meaning. The shift from a defensive to an optimistic stance allows them to engage with the world and their relationships in healthier, more fulfilling ways.

In conclusion, reinforcing positive beliefs in therapy is truly about planting seeds of possibility in the fertile ground of an individual's psyche. It's about reminding them of the innate strengths they possess and helping them transform these into guiding principles. In doing so, therapists assist individuals not just in healing, but in rebuilding their lives in a way that celebrates their resilience and potential.

CHAPTER 12

SAFETY ISSUES IN CPT

In the delicate process of Cognitive Processing Therapy (CPT), safety stands as an unwavering cornerstone. As therapists guide patients through the challenging landscapes of trauma and memory, the potential for crisis situations looms. It's imperative to establish a robust safety plan that respects the patient's pace and emotional limits. Managing the fine line between therapeutic exposure and overwhelming distress requires a deft hand; therapists must continuously balance encouraging patients to face their trauma with ensuring their emotional and psychological safety.

Proactive strategies not only prevent crises but also empower patients to reclaim a sense of control. By infusing therapy with compassion and vigilance, we create a sanctuary where healing can truly begin, opening pathways for growth while safeguarding the emotional well-being of those we serve.

In navigating the delicate balance between confronting trauma and safeguarding emotional well-being, therapists must remain attuned to each patient's readiness to process painful memories. Research in trauma-informed care highlights the importance of pacing during therapy, acknowledging that pushing too quickly into trauma processing can overwhelm the client and potentially lead to retraumatization. By adopting a patient-centered approach, therapists ensure that patients have a sense of agency and control over the pace at which they engage with their trauma. This approach not only promotes safety but also fosters trust, which is essential for creating the strong therapeutic alliance necessary for healing. The goal is to empower patients to face their past at a pace that respects their emotional capacity, allowing them to gradually integrate their traumatic experiences without overwhelming their psychological defenses.

Furthermore, proactive strategies in therapy, such as grounding techniques, mindfulness practices, and emotional regulation skills, are critical tools that help patients manage distressing emotions in the moment. These techniques are rooted in cognitive-behavioral and mindfulness-based therapies, both of which have demonstrated efficacy in helping individuals cope with the aftereffects of trauma. Grounding exercises, for example, help patients stay connected to the present moment, preventing them from becoming overwhelmed by flashbacks or intrusive memories. By equipping patients with these practical tools, therapists not only enhance their immediate coping abilities but also support their long-term emotional resilience. In doing so, therapy becomes a space of both challenge and safety, where patients can begin to reclaim their sense of control and rebuild their lives from a place of empowerment.

Handling Crisis Situations

In the therapeutic journey, crises can emerge unpredictably, thrusting both the therapist and the patient into challenging terrain. When it comes to handling crisis situations in the context of Cognitive Processing Therapy (CPT), preparation is paramount. The goal is to create a pathway through tumultuous times, ensuring both safety and progress in healing. At the heart of managing these situations is a blend of awareness, proactive planning, and adaptive responses.

The nature of trauma and its pervasive impact means that crises are not only about the here and now but can also be rooted in past wounds. A crisis may stem from the patient's environment—such as relationships or external stresses—or from the therapeutic work itself, as patients confront traumatic memories and potentially destabilizing emotions. It's essential that health professionals recognize the nuanced triggers and remain vigilant, while sustaining a grounding, reassuring presence for their patients.

Understanding the particularities of each patient is critical. No two crisis situations are the same, for they are interwoven with the unique histories and sensitivities of those experiencing them. Empathy and attentive listening become indispensable tools in discerning the layers of a crisis. They allow the therapist to navigate the unfolding situation with gentle precision—balancing between addressing immediate safety concerns and encouraging the process of emotional exploration that CPT aims to foster.

Preparation includes establishing clear crisis management protocols well ahead of therapy sessions. These protocols should provide therapists with guidelines for responding effectively, whether that means having emergency contact information at the ready or collaborating with other mental health services when more intensive support is required. Moreover, therapists should discuss potential crisis scenarios with their patients early on, crafting a shared understanding and strategy for what to do should a crisis arise. This proactive stance not only equips patients with coping mechanisms but also fosters a collaborative therapeutic alliance grounded in trust and mutual respect.

Grounding techniques play an instrumental role in crisis management within CPT. These techniques help individuals stay connected to the present moment, mitigating overwhelming feelings that can hijack their sense of stability. Such techniques might include mindfulness practices, sensory reinforcements, or simple breathing exercises—each tailored to comfort and redirect the mind during distressing moments. Utilizing these strategies regularly can bolster a patient's resilience, enhancing their capacity to manage crises when they arise.

Additionally, the role of self-regulation cannot be overstated. Learning to recognize and modulate emotions is a foundational skill in dealing with crises. For therapists, modeling healthy emotional regulation is just as vital as teaching it. By exemplifying calmness and patience, therapists provide a living example for patients, showing that it is possible to steer through the storm without becoming engulfed by it.

Every plan needs flexibility—an ability to pivot in response to unexpected developments. During a crisis, adapting plans to meet the immediate needs of the patient is crucial. This might involve temporarily altering the focus of therapy sessions, offering more frequent sessions, or incorporating additional therapeutic modalities to support stabilization. As stability is regained, the focus can slowly shift back to the core goals of CPT, always aligning with the patient's pace and readiness.

Support networks are invaluable during crises. Encouraging patients to identify and lean on trusted individuals from their lives, whether friends, family members, or community groups, provides additional layers of support. These networks are essential faucets of assistance during times when the therapist isn't readily available. Incorporating these supports within the treatment plan can enhance the patient's safety and resilience.

It's equally important to attend to the therapist's well-being amid managing crisis situations. Handling someone else's crisis can echo resonantly within the therapist, potentially leading to secondary stress or burnout. Therefore, therapists should engage in regular self-care practices and seek supervision or consultation when needed. This reflection and support not only safeguard the therapist but also enrich their capacity to be fully present and effective for their patients.

Therapists must remember that handling crisis situations in CPT is as much about creativity as it is about steadfastness. Every instance of crisis presents an opportunity for breakthroughs and deeper understanding. By approaching these situations not as detours, but as integral components of the healing journey, therapists empower their patients to transform moments of crisis into pivotal stepping stones towards recovery.

Crisis management in CPT thus becomes a dance of initiative, empathy, and adaptability, deeply rooted in evidence-based practice yet sensitive to the dynamic intricacies of human experience. With the right strategies and a compassionate presence, therapists can guide their patients through the most challenging of times, fostering growth, resilience, and a profound sense of empowerment that extends beyond the therapy room.

Safety Planning

Safety planning is a vital, non-negotiable component of Cognitive Processing Therapy (CPT) that anchors the therapeutic process in a foundation of security and trust. For healthcare providers and mental health professionals, understanding the intricacies of safety planning within the CPT framework is indispensable. This process not only safeguards patient's immediate well-being but also facilitates the therapeutic journey towards healing and recovery. Safety planning is a proactive strategy designed to mitigate risk, manage crises, and ensure that patients have the necessary resources to protect themselves outside of therapy sessions.

The cornerstone of effective safety planning involves a detailed understanding of the client's specific risks and triggers. It's a personalized plan, tailored to the unique history and current circumstances of the patient. This necessitates an in-depth assessment phase where therapists identify potential situations that could compromise the patient's safety.

Employing compassionate inquiry, therapists can discern patterns and anticipate challenges, ensuring that the plan is both comprehensive and culturally sensitive. This personalized approach empowers clients, instilling a sense of agency and preparedness in potentially destabilizing situations.

An empathetic, collaborative approach to safety planning enhances the therapeutic alliance. Patients are often in vulnerable positions, and by engaging them directly in the safety planning process, therapists reinforce a sense of partnership and mutual trust. This partnership is critical, as patients are more inclined to adhere to a plan they've actively co-created. Open communication and transparency foster an environment where clients feel heard and understood, reducing anxiety and increasing their confidence in the plan.

Safety plans are not static documents; they're dynamic frameworks that require continual assessment and adjustment. As therapy progresses and patients develop new coping strategies and resilience, the safety plan should evolve. Regularly revisiting and modifying the plan in response to changing needs and risks is crucial. This iterative process reflects a commitment to the patient's growth, adapting to their journey towards recovery and reclaiming their autonomy.

The inclusion of specific, actionable strategies in the safety plan is essential. This might include identifying supportive contacts who can be reached in moments of crisis, outlining safe spaces where the patient can go if they feel threatened, and establishing a clear, step-by-step process for seeking help. Concrete strategies provide clarity and guidance, reducing the likelihood of panic and confusion in critical moments.

Patients gain confidence and reassurance, knowing they have a clear roadmap to follow.

Therapists should incorporate psychoeducation as part of the safety planning process. Educating patients about their physiological and psychological responses to trauma can demystify their experiences and normalize their reactions. Knowledge is power, and understanding the roots and manifestations of fear and distress can be transformative. This educational component empowers patients, providing them with the tools to anticipate reactions and implement prevention techniques effectively.

Mindfulness and grounding exercises can also play a significant role in safety planning. Skills such as deep breathing, progressive muscle relaxation, and grounding techniques empower patients to regulate emotional arousal and maintain a sense of calm during distressing situations. These techniques can be life-saving tools in preventing the escalation of fear or panic, allowing the patient to remain in control of their reactions and the situation at hand.

In some cases, medication management may be necessary as part of a comprehensive safety plan. Collaboration with psychiatrists or primary care physicians can facilitate a multidisciplinary approach ensuring that any pharmacological interventions support the patient's therapeutic goals. It's critical that any medicinal strategies are seamlessly integrated into the overall plan and are carefully monitored to prevent potential side effects or dependency issues.

Importantly, safety planning must take into account the potential for digital threats, especially in an increasingly interconnected world. Patients may face harassment or threats via social media or other online platforms. As part of safety planning, therapists can assist patients in managing their digital presence, implementing privacy settings, and recognizing online risks. Educating patients about online safety can fortify their defenses against the unique perils of the digital age.

Ultimately, the goal of safety planning within CPT is to create a robust framework that supports patient healing without exposing them to undue harm. It is about balancing the need for therapeutic exposure and processing of trauma material with the necessity of maintaining patient safety. A well-crafted safety plan aligns with the primary therapeutic goal of CPT—helping patients reclaim their lives and mental space from the shadow of past traumas.

This reflects a commitment to fostering resilience and hope, guiding individuals toward a future where they feel secure, empowered, and in control. By applying a meticulous and compassionate approach to safety planning, therapists not only protect their patients but also pave the way for enduring therapeutic success. The meticulous identification of potential threats, co-creation of actionable strategies, and flexibility in plan adaptation ensures that safety planning is not just a preventative measure, but a powerful catalyst for transformative change.

Balancing Exposure in Therapy

In the realm of Cognitive Processing Therapy (CPT), the concept of exposure is vital yet delicate. It's about meeting the trauma and not letting it dictate the terms of engagement. Exposure in therapy aims to help individuals confront and process their trauma in a safe and controlled environment. The balance here is crucial, as the therapeutic process demands a harmony that nurtures growth while safeguarding the client's psychological well-being. The notion isn't just to relive the trauma but to face it progressively, with the ultimate goal of integrating past experiences in a way that promotes healing.

Safe exposure in therapy begins with the client's preparedness. Therapists must ensure that the groundwork is securely laid out through comprehensive initial assessments and the creation of a therapeutic alliance. Only then can exposure techniques be employed effectively to navigate the emotional and cognitive landscapes shaped by trauma.

It's essential to calibrate this process meticulously. Too much exposure too quickly can re-traumatize individuals, while insufficient exposure may hinder the healing journey.

The art of balancing exposure lies in understanding the client's current coping mechanisms, resilience, and readiness to engage deeply with their trauma narrative. Therapists must tune into these variables, adapting their approach based on ongoing evaluations. Engaging clients in their trauma narratives requires fostering an environment where disclosure feels not only permissible but empowering. This involves guiding them through the process with empathy, every step of the way.

- Start where the client is: Understanding their starting point can make all the difference. Identify their existing strategies for coping and build upon them.
- Tailor the approach: No two clients are the same—differences in past experiences, cultural

backgrounds, and personal beliefs shape how trauma is perceived and processed.

- Set realistic goals: Aim for achievable milestones that reflect both the client's aspirations and therapeutic plausibility.

Motivation plays a significant role in this balance. As practitioners guide their clients through exposure activities, emphasizing the therapeutic goal of reclaiming autonomy over one's mind and emotions becomes critical. When clients understand and believe in the purpose behind their actions, their engagement deepens, allowing for a more fruitful therapy journey. Thus, exposure becomes not just an intervention but a pathway to resilience.

Client safety is paramount. Effective exposure therapy doesn't rush the client past their limits. Instead, it acknowledges these boundaries while gently challenging them, ensuring the client never feels cornered. Such an approach requires continual dialogue, where therapists invite feedback and adjust strategies, reinforcing the collaborative nature of the therapy.

Here, the therapist's skill in implementing adaptive strategies is tested. Weaving encouragement with caution, they must remain attentive to their client's responses during exposure tasks, ready to pivot based on emerging needs. This might mean pausing to process emotions or redefining the pace of therapy. Flexibility is the cornerstone, guiding the client safely through their exposure work without the risk of triggering adverse effects.

Therapists also need to be vigilant of avoidance techniques clients might use to shy away from the painful truths of their narratives. The task is to identify such patterns gently and redefine them into opportunities for therapeutic engagement. Addressing avoidance involves opening channels for dialogue about fears and discomforts related to exposure tasks. This can highlight moments of self-sabotage, turning them into breakthroughs rather than setbacks.

1. Detect avoidance: Listen actively for signs of hesitation or reluctance.
2. Engage in compassionate confrontation: Address avoidance patterns with empathy and understanding.
3. Transform willingness into strength: Foster a supportive atmosphere where the client's readiness can blossom into resilience.

Ultimately, the cognitive restructuring that is central to CPT benefits from a well-orchestrated exposure process. This balance evolves into a dance— where therapists and clients move in a dynamic exchange of challenge and support. At the core, successful exposure strategies in therapy are those that empower clients, allowing them to move towards a narrative of hope and transformation.

Balancing exposure in therapy reinforces the importance of structure and spontaneity within the therapeutic environment. It reflects the fundamental belief that past traumas don't have to constrain the future. When handled deftly, exposure work in CPT can be a catalyst for profound change, where clients emerge not only with newfound understanding but with a reinvigorated sense of self-empowerment. Through careful navigation of exposure, therapists can assist clients in embracing the breadth of their experiences with clarity and confidence, culminating in healing that is both authentic and enduring.

CHAPTER 13

CPT FOR DIVERSE POPULATIONS

In any therapeutic setting, acknowledging and embracing diversity isn't just an ideal—it's a necessity. Cognitive Processing Therapy (CPT) must adapt to the rich tapestry of human experiences shaped by culture, ethnicity, gender identity, and more. Effective practitioners understand that cultural sensitivity is crucial, not as a checkbox, but as a cornerstone of genuine healing. This chapter considers how therapists can flexibly tailor CPT techniques to resonate with individuals from diverse backgrounds, ensuring that interventions align with each person's unique cultural narratives and lived experiences. Just as no two traumas are identical, the cultural contexts in which people endure and recover from trauma differ, requiring a nuanced approach. Addressing unique needs involves not only adapting language and techniques but also actively listening and learning, showing empathy for paths that might differ from one's own. Practitioners are called to examine their assumptions and biases, fostering an environment where every individual feels seen, heard, and understood. In doing so, they facilitate not just recovery, but empowerment, honoring the resilience that diverse communities bring to the journey of healing. By making these considered adaptations, we don't just offer treatment; we offer a means to reclaim one's narrative from the shadows of trauma and illuminate a path forward.

Cultural Sensitivity

Cultural sensitivity in Cognitive Processing Therapy (CPT) is not simply an add-on but an essential core element. In working with diverse populations, therapists must be acutely aware that culture shapes an individual's experiences and perceptions of trauma. It defines what is considered traumatic and influences the ways in which people cope with and express distress. Thus, understanding cultural diversity isn't merely beneficial, it's a necessity for effective therapy.

Central to cultural sensitivity is acknowledging and respecting the client's cultural background. For clients from different cultural backgrounds, PTSD symptoms may manifest in ways that don't align with traditional Western diagnostic criteria. As practitioners, it's crucial to listen deeply and adapt treatment plans in ways that honor these cultural differences.

This adaptability fosters a stronger therapeutic alliance, as clients feel seen and understood in the fullness of their identity.

Practitioners should strive to build their cultural competence continuously. This ongoing journey towards understanding diverse cultures helps bridge potential gaps between therapist and client. It's about cultivating an environment where clients from all backgrounds feel safe to express and explore the impact of their cultural identity within the therapeutic process. By doing so, therapists reinforce a message of inclusivity and respect.

One effective approach to integrating cultural sensitivity in CPT is through personalized assessments. These assessments categorize and evaluate cultural dimensions that may influence trauma responses and therapeutic engagement. By understanding individuals' cultural contexts, therapists can tailor interventions to meet clients where they are, using language, metaphors, and perspectives that resonate deeply with them.

Cultural humility goes hand in hand with cultural sensitivity. It's about remaining open to learning from clients about their cultural worldviews, acknowledging the limits of your own cultural understanding. Therapists should recognize that they are not the ultimate authority on a client's experiences. This humility fosters mutual respect and creates a therapeutic space where honesty and authenticity can thrive.

Moreover, cultural beliefs often play a significant role in shaping a person's understanding and expression of trauma. It's crucial to engage in discussions about these beliefs, as they can either act as sources of resilience or as barriers to healing. By validating these beliefs and exploring their context, therapists can guide clients in integrating their cultural strengths into their healing journeys.

Acknowledging cultural taboos is equally important. In some cultures, discussing mental health issues is frowned upon, and PTSD symptoms might be attributed to spiritual causes or seen as a sign of personal weakness. Understanding these perspectives allows therapists to approach such subjects with sensitivity and care, facilitating dialogues that respect the client's beliefs while gently introducing new therapeutic perspectives.

Another pivotal aspect of cultural sensitivity in CPT is the adaptation of psychoeducational materials. Materials should reflect the cultural narratives and values of the populations they serve. This involves using examples and situations that are culturally relevant and relatable to the client, fostering a sense of connection and understanding from the outset of therapy.

For therapists working with refugees or immigrants, being culturally sensitive means understanding the significant impact of acculturation stress and historical trauma. Many clients from these backgrounds carry the psychological weight of displacement and the loss of familiar cultural systems. Exploring these themes within CPT can aid in addressing not only trauma but also auxiliary stressors related to adaptation and identity transformation in a new cultural context.

Language is a fundamental component of cultural sensitivity. Being able to communicate in a client's preferred language or utilizing competent interpreters is vital. Miscommunication or lack of understanding can create additional barriers, further alienating the client and undermining the therapy process. Non-verbal communication should also be considered, as gestures, eye contact, and body language vary significantly across cultures.

Therapists should also be mindful of their own cultural biases and how these might affect their perceptions and interactions within therapy sessions. Reflective practice and supervision are valuable tools that help therapists recognize and deconstruct these biases. This self-awareness is pivotal in avoiding potentially harmful assumptions and fostering a practice that is genuinely client-centered.

Involving community leaders and utilizing culturally relevant resources could also enhance cultural sensitivity in CPT. Collaborating with figures who hold cultural authority can help legitimize the therapeutic process in the eyes of the client. This partnership can demystify therapy and make mental health care more approachable within the community it serves.

Cultural sensitivity does not mean compromising the core tenets of CPT but rather adapting its application to ensure its effectiveness across varied cultural settings. This includes being willing to modify the therapy approach and possibly the structure of sessions to align better with cultural expectations and norms. Such flexibility demonstrates respect and commitment to truly understanding and serving the client's best interests.

Ultimately, cultural sensitivity in CPT empowers therapists to not only understand but celebrate the rich tapestry of human diversity. By embracing cultural differences, therapists can provide more compassionate, effective care that fosters healing in ways that are congruent with each client's unique cultural narrative. This process requires ongoing reflection and dedication to learning, ensuring that therapy remains a space of growth and understanding for all involved.

Adapting Techniques

In the nuanced landscape of Cognitive Processing Therapy (CPT), one size doesn't fit all. Adapting techniques is crucial to ensure the therapy resonates with the diverse populations we encounter in our practice. As mental health professionals, we strive to bridge the gap between evidence- based methods and the lived experiences of our clients. This means tailoring CPT strategies to not only align with cultural backgrounds but also to meet the unique psychological needs and circumstances of each individual.

Understanding cultural context is the first step in adaptation. Different cultural groups have varied ways of interpreting and expressing distress, which might influence their engagement in therapy. A person from a collectivist culture, for instance, might emphasize family or community values more than individualistic goals. Recognizing and integrating these cultural nuances into therapy not only enhances therapeutic alliance but also makes interventions like identifying and challenging maladaptive thoughts more relatable and effective.

Rather than imposing a rigid structure, therapists can adapt therapeutic interventions to honor clients' values and belief systems. This might mean using culturally relevant metaphors or analogies to explain CPT concepts. Additionally, some clients may benefit from adjustments in how emotional processing is handled, respecting cultural norms around emotional expression or resilience. Customizing therapeutic language and techniques in this way helps in fostering a supportive environment where clients feel understood and respected.

Language can be another important aspect of adapting CPT. For clients who speak multiple languages or have limited proficiency in the primary language of therapy, it's essential to ensure that communication is both clear and meaningful. This might involve the use of bilingual materials, interpreters, or even culturally specific idioms that convey critical concepts in a more graspable way. When clients feel they can communicate their thoughts and feelings without the barrier of language, the depth of therapy can be profoundly enhanced.

It's also important to consider the socio-economic and systemic factors that shape a person's experience of trauma and their response to therapy. Economic hardships, exposure to violence, and historical trauma due to systemic oppression can significantly impact mental health.

Acknowledging these factors in therapy, and adjusting the focus and pace of CPT accordingly, helps address root causes and provides clients with more sustainable coping strategies. Therapists can work to empower individuals by integrating strength-based approaches that build on their existing resilience and community resources.

Beyond cultural and linguistic adaptations, therapists should be attentive to developmental differences, particularly when working with children or adolescents. Younger clients may require modified versions of standard CPT exercises. Employing creative techniques, such as story-telling, drawing, or role-play, can make complex concepts more accessible and engaging. Involving the family in therapy can also provide crucial support for younger clients, reinforcing new ways of thinking and behaving outside therapy sessions.

Adapting techniques also involves being flexible with the structure and pacing of therapy. For some clients, adherence to a strict session timeline might be counterproductive, especially if additional time is needed to develop trust or process difficult emotions. Flexibility could mean allowing more time for certain activities or revisiting specific aspects of the therapy that need further attention. This adaptability ensures that therapy progresses in a manner that's most beneficial for the client.

It's important to remember the evolving nature of trauma therapy itself. New research and feedback from diverse client groups can inform innovative approaches to CPT. Staying updated with current findings, and being open to changing one's methods accordingly, allows therapists to offer the most effective and compassionate care possible.

Finally, the process of adapting CPT techniques requires ongoing education and self-reflection from therapists. Professionals should engage in continual learning about the cultural, social, and individual factors that can influence therapy outcomes. Regular supervision and peer consultation can provide valuable perspectives and guidance, helping therapists maintain a high standard of care for all clients.

In essence, adapting techniques within the framework of CPT for diverse populations is an act of profound respect and empathy. It's about honoring the person behind the symptoms and offering a therapeutic approach that not only addresses their trauma but also celebrates their strengths and potential for healing. By doing so, we not only contribute to their recovery but also enrich our own professional practice.

Addressing Unique Needs

In Cognitive Processing Therapy (CPT), understanding and addressing the unique needs of diverse populations is vital. This section delves into the complexities of tailoring therapeutic techniques to fit individual cultural contexts, identities, and experiences. The goal is to provide health care providers, clinicians, and mental health professionals with the insights needed to modify their approaches in a way that is both sensitive and effective.

Every individual brings their own cultural backdrop and personal history to therapy. Recognizing and respecting this diversity is not just ethical; it's practical. When therapists incorporate cultural sensitivity into their practice, they create an environment that feels safe and welcoming for all clients. This can promote deeper engagement and openness in the therapeutic process. By acknowledging cultural differences, therapists can avoid misinterpretations that may arise from culturally specific expressions of distress.

Addressing unique needs often begins with understanding cultural values and belief systems. For instance, some cultures may view mental health differently, affecting how clients perceive their symptoms and treatment. By being informed about these diverse perspectives, therapists can communicate more effectively and adjust their strategies accordingly. Practitioners must not assume universality in experiences but instead, consider how culture shapes an individual's understanding of trauma and healing.

Language barriers can also pose significant challenges in therapy. Using professional interpreters or seeking resources in a client's native language can help bridge these gaps. It's crucial for therapists to ensure that the expression and nuances of emotional experiences are accurately conveyed. Miscommunication can lead to misunderstandings or missed nuances in a client's narrative that are essential for cognitive processing.

Besides language, religious beliefs and spiritual practices also significantly influence how individuals process trauma. Recognizing and integrating these elements into therapy can enhance the therapeutic relationship. By working collaboratively with clients to understand their spiritual and religious frameworks, therapists can identify practices or rituals that may support the therapeutic process, fostering a sense of resilience and community.

Gender identity and sexual orientation are other facets where unique needs become apparent. Creating an inclusive and affirming space is crucial. Therapists should be acutely aware of the potential for systemic discrimination that these clients might face and be prepared to address how such experiences compound trauma. Training in LGBTQ+ issues and adopting a stance of affirmation are essential for therapists working with these populations.

The intersectionality of various identities can create layers of complexity in understanding and addressing trauma. Acknowledging how race, gender, class, and ability intersect in a client's life is necessary for effective treatment. These intersections can influence not only how trauma is experienced but also how healing is approached. Culturally informed assessments and interventions help in navigating these complex layers with empathy and precision.

For individuals from refugee or immigrant backgrounds, there are added layers of complexity surrounding displacement, acculturation stress, and sometimes, pre-migration trauma. It's crucial for therapists to recognize these additional stressors and the role they play in the client's current mental health status. Providing resources that help navigate the challenges of a new environment can be an integral part of the therapeutic process.

Socioeconomic status also plays a role in how accessible and feasible therapy is for clients. Therapists should consider the financial and logistical barriers that might prevent clients from fully engaging in therapy. Sliding scale fees, flexible scheduling, and locating additional community resources can help overcome some of these barriers, promoting equal access to therapeutic benefits for all.

Furthermore, addressing past negative experiences with mental health systems is essential for some clients. Many individuals from marginalized communities may carry a distrust of mental health services due to historical mistreatment. Building trust requires time, transparency, and consistency. Therapists should acknowledge this history and involve clients collaboratively in the treatment planning process to enhance empowerment and engagement.

Incorporating trauma-informed care principles is particularly beneficial when addressing the unique needs of diverse populations. These principles remind therapists to prioritize a client's safety and trust while understanding the impact of trauma. It requires a shift from asking "What is wrong with you?" to "What happened to you?" This reframing is supportive and less re-traumatizing, allowing the client to explore their past without shame or judgment.

In conclusion, addressing unique needs in CPT is an ongoing process of cultural competence, empathy, and adaptability. It is about meeting clients where they are, not just in terms of their trauma, but in the totality of their identity. By doing so, therapists foster a space where healing is not a one- size-fits-all experience but a personalized journey towards reclaiming mental space and wellbeing. This work empowers professionals to become allies in their clients' lives, walking alongside them as they navigate the complexities of their healing journey.

CHAPTER 14

SPECIAL CONSIDERATIONS IN CPT

When working with Cognitive Processing Therapy (CPT), it's crucial to understand the nuanced needs that arise when treating individuals with co- occurring disorders, comorbidities, and complex trauma. Each patient's experience is unique, and their therapeutic journey should be, too.

Adjustments may need to be made in the standard CPT protocol to accommodate these special considerations, ensuring that treatment is both effective and empathetic. Co-occurring disorders often require integrated therapeutic approaches, marrying CPT with other interventions to address a full spectrum of mental health needs. Similarly, the presence of complex traumas can call for a more flexible pacing in therapy sessions, allowing for the patient's safety and comfort. Therapists must be attuned to these dynamics, using their skills and judgment to tailor the therapy process while keeping the core principles of CPT intact. This responsiveness not only fosters healing but also empowers patients to navigate their recovery with greater agency and resilience.

When working with individuals who have co-occurring disorders and complex trauma, it is essential for therapists to recognize the intricate interplay between different mental health challenges. Research has shown that individuals with both trauma and mental health conditions such as depression, anxiety, or substance use disorders often face compounded struggles, requiring a more holistic and flexible approach to treatment. For example, trauma can exacerbate symptoms of anxiety or depression, while substance use may serve as a coping mechanism to numb emotional pain. In these cases, combining CPT with other evidence-based treatments like Dialectical Behavior Therapy (DBT) or Motivational Interviewing can create a more comprehensive therapeutic plan. These integrated approaches help address the full scope of the patient's needs, allowing for better outcomes. Furthermore, providing a trauma-sensitive environment that acknowledges the patient's past experiences with mental health challenges can create a safe space where they feel understood, reducing the likelihood of disengagement and increasing the effectiveness of therapy.

Co-occurring Disorders

When working with individuals who have experienced trauma, it is essential to consider the complexity added by co-occurring disorders. Many patients seeking Cognitive Processing Therapy (CPT) for PTSD may also struggle with other mental health issues such as anxiety, depression, substance use disorders, or personality disorders.

Recognizing the presence of these disorders is crucial for effective treatment. They can significantly impact the course and outcome of therapy if not adequately addressed at the onset.

In situations where PTSD coexists with other mental health conditions, a tailored approach becomes necessary. Dual diagnosis can complicate symptom presentation, making it harder for clinicians to discern the root problem. For instance, someone struggling with both PTSD and a substance use disorder may use substances as a coping mechanism for trauma-related distress. This can cloud the PTSD symptoms, complicating both diagnosis and treatment.

As such, clinicians must remain vigilant in their assessments while remaining attuned to the dynamic interaction between PTSD symptoms and those of co-occurring disorders.

Understanding the intersecting symptoms of PTSD and other disorders helps guide treatment planning. Cognitive distortions—a key focus of CPT—may be influenced by co-occurring disorders, necessitating adjustments in the standard approach to cognitive processing. For example, depression can exacerbate negative thought patterns, while anxiety might amplify avoidance behaviors. By identifying and addressing these interlinked manifestations, therapists can more effectively target the beliefs and behaviors hindering recovery.

It's important to foster a therapeutic environment that recognizes the challenges posed by these overlapping conditions. The therapist-patient alliance must be built on empathy, understanding, and openness. Patients often face stigma related to their co-occurring disorders, making it vital to address any misconceptions they may hold. Education around the interaction between their PTSD and co-occurring disorders can empower patients to engage fully in the therapeutic process, laying the groundwork for substantial progress.

Therapists should remain flexible, revisiting and revising treatment goals as necessary to accommodate the shifting landscape of patients' needs. Regularly assessing the presence and severity of co-occurring symptoms throughout the course of therapy allows for dynamic treatment adaptations. Such adjustments can include integrating elements of other therapeutic modalities, like motivational interviewing for substance use or mindfulness for anxiety, creating a more holistic and responsive intervention strategy.

Research indicates that simultaneous treatment of PTSD and co-occurring disorders can be highly effective. However, one must approach each case uniquely, considering the patient's personal history, preferences, and specific symptomatology. For instance, prioritizing one disorder over the others may be beneficial in certain contexts, while an integrative approach that addresses both simultaneously might be more appropriate in others.

While dealing with these complexities, maintaining the integrity of the CPT model is vital. Yet, flexibility within the framework is necessary to address individual differences and co-morbid presentations effectively. In practice, this might involve introducing additional sessions that focus specifically on symptoms or integrating supplemental therapeutic techniques that target the accompanying disorder directly.

The challenge for mental health providers is not only to recognize and treat the primary symptoms of PTSD but also to be strategic in navigating the terrain of co-occurring disorders. The need for interdisciplinary collaboration can't be understated; partnering with other specialists within psychiatry, primary care, substance abuse services, and broader mental health supports can provide patients with the comprehensive care they require.

Addressing co-occurring disorders is not merely an adjunct to trauma therapy; it is a core component of effective treatment for many patients. Ensuring that treatment plans meet the nuanced needs of these patients requires a steadfast commitment to comprehensive care. By prioritizing a holistic, individualized approach that champions patient strengths and empowers them to tackle each aspect of their mental health, providers can catalyze profound healing and transformation.

Ultimately, our goal as mental health professionals is to foster an environment where patients feel supported and understood, not only in addressing their PTSD but also in conquering the additional hurdles presented by co-occurring disorders. In doing so, we pave the way for more meaningful and lasting recovery, offering a path to regaining autonomy and a higher quality of life.

A key aspect of navigating co-occurring disorders is recognizing the complex ways in which multiple conditions can interact and amplify each other. For example, PTSD and depression frequently coexist, with symptoms of one exacerbating the other, creating a vicious cycle that is difficult to break. Studies have shown that when PTSD and depression are treated together, rather than in isolation, outcomes improve significantly, as addressing both conditions simultaneously allows for a more comprehensive understanding of the patient's struggles. By providing integrated care that targets both the trauma and the depressive symptoms, therapists can help patients interrupt this cycle, reducing the overall burden of mental health challenges and improving the quality of their lives. This integrated approach is especially important as many individuals with co-occurring disorders may not seek help for all of their conditions, further complicating the treatment process.

Furthermore, the importance of a trauma-informed approach cannot be overstated when working with individuals who have co-occurring disorders. Trauma-informed care goes beyond simply addressing trauma symptoms; it reshapes the entire therapeutic environment to recognize the pervasive impact of trauma on a person's life. This approach promotes safety, trustworthiness, and empowerment, all of which are foundational to effective treatment. Research shows that when mental health providers apply trauma-informed principles across all aspects of care, patients experience lower rates of disengagement and higher satisfaction with treatment. For individuals with co-occurring disorders, the trauma-informed framework ensures that each professional interaction is sensitive to the patient's past experiences and current vulnerabilities, facilitating an atmosphere of healing that promotes long-term recovery.

In the context of interdisciplinary collaboration, communication among providers is essential to ensure that treatment remains coordinated and that each professional is aware of the patient's progress. A recent study highlighted that integrated care teams, where providers from various disciplines communicate regularly, have been shown to enhance the effectiveness of treatment for individuals with complex mental health issues. By sharing insights and expertise, therapists, psychiatrists, addiction counselors, and primary care physicians can better align their approaches, prevent potential conflicts between medications or treatment methods, and ensure that all aspects of a patient's mental health are addressed. This holistic care model reduces the risk of fragmented care, ensuring that patients benefit from a more unified treatment plan that increases the likelihood of sustained recovery.

Finally, empowering patients to take an active role in their treatment is crucial for fostering lasting change. Research in motivational interviewing has demonstrated that when patients are encouraged to set their own goals and make decisions about their treatment, they are more likely to stay engaged and motivated throughout the healing process. This empowerment is especially vital for individuals with co-occurring disorders, as they may have developed a sense of helplessness or resignation in the face of their complex challenges. By involving patients in their care, mental health professionals can help them rediscover their agency, giving them the tools to not only cope with their symptoms but to build a future that is not defined by their struggles. This approach fosters a sense of autonomy, dignity, and hope, creating a foundation for profound, long-term healing.

Adjustments for Comorbidities

In the complex terrain of Cognitive Processing Therapy (CPT), addressing comorbidities—conditions that occur simultaneously with PTSD—is both a critical challenge and an opportunity for holistic healing. Effective therapy recognizes the multifaceted nature of an individual's health, understanding that disorders such as depression, anxiety, or substance use do not occur in isolation but often interplay with

PTSD, affecting the therapeutic process. Thus, the task at hand for clinicians is to customize CPT to respect and incorporate these complexities rather than attempt to compartmentalize them.

The first adjustment comes from acknowledging that the presence of comorbidities can alter the manifestation of PTSD symptoms. For instance, in patients with concurrent major depressive disorder, the cognitive distortions and negative beliefs central to CPT might be more entrenched. Depressive features can color the patient's trauma narrative with a lens of hopelessness or self-reproach. Therapists must therefore be prepared to adapt interventions, perhaps spending additional time on cognitive restructuring exercises to challenge pervasive feelings of inadequacy or guilt before delving deeper into specific PTSD-related cognitions.

Anxiety disorders, another frequent comorbid condition, demand a balanced calibration within the CPT framework. Anxiety can exacerbate avoidance behaviors, a core symptom of PTSD, impeding progress in therapy where confronting avoided memories and situations is necessary. In such cases, pacing is everything. Therapists need to strategically introduce exposure elements in therapy, ensuring the patient feels equipped with skills to manage anxiety. Graduated exposure and the incorporation of relaxation techniques are crucial adjustments that can enable the patient to engage with trauma processing more constructively.

Moreover, substance use disorders, which often co-occur with PTSD, require careful navigation within CPT. Substance use can be a maladaptive coping mechanism to manage trauma-related distress, necessitating an integrative approach that addresses both the behavioral patterns of addiction and the cognitive aspects of PTSD. Here, inter-disciplinary collaboration is vital. Coordinating with addiction specialists or implementing concurrent treatment models can ensure that CPT is not hindered by ongoing substance use, providing a comprehensive support framework for the patient.

Adjustments in CPT for patients with comorbidities also encompass practical modifications. For instance, structuring sessions that interlace cognitive behavioral strategies specific to secondary disorders—such as mindfulness-based interventions for co-existing anxiety or motivational interviewing for substance use—into the CPT framework can create a seamless therapeutic experience. This integrative approach not only addresses the breadth of the patient's mental health needs but also enhances their engagement and buy-in to the therapeutic process.

Furthermore, the clinician's sensitivity to the presence of complex trauma, often characterized by multiple traumas and a backdrop of adverse childhood experiences, is essential. Here, the therapeutic pathways must be even more flexible. Patients with complex trauma can present with a range of comorbidities that require more nuanced therapeutic approaches

—potentially slowing the pacing of CPT and taking care to build a robust therapeutic alliance before delving into trauma-focused work.

Empathy and adaptability in therapy are foundational when dealing with comorbid conditions. Therapists must not only recognize the barriers these conditions create but also view them as a compass that guides personalized therapy. This entails a shift from rigidity to flexibility in the therapeutic agenda. Therapists might find it beneficial to include more psychoeducational components, helping patients understand the interplay of their comorbid conditions with PTSD, thus fostering a greater sense of control and self-efficacy.

Adjustments for comorbidities don't stop at treatment techniques; they extend to the therapeutic relationship itself. Building a steadfast alliance is imperative, as is ensuring the patient feels seen and heard beyond their

PTSD symptomatology. Regular check-ins about how the therapy aligns with the patient's goals can inform necessary adjustments. Validation of the hardships imposed by comorbid conditions is a key thread that weaves trust into the therapeutic process.

Ultimately, the adjustments for comorbidities in CPT are not mere tweaks but encompass a paradigm that embraces complexity, promotes resilience, and advocates for a patient-centered approach. By tailoring treatment to meet the intertwining needs of each individual, providers can facilitate a therapeutic journey that acknowledges the whole person, guiding them toward reclaiming their mental space with newfound clarity and empowerment.

This dynamic, adaptable approach to CPT empowers health care providers, researchers, and mental health professionals to offer compelling, empathetic interventions that strengthen therapeutic efficacy. In essence, it's a collaborative effort to build pathways to recovery that honor each person's unique journey, contributing significantly to the overarching goal of reclaiming time and mental space in the realm of PTSD and beyond.

Considerations for Complex Trauma

When working with individuals experiencing complex trauma, it's vital to acknowledge the multifaceted nature of their experiences. Complex trauma often involves repeated or prolonged trauma and can occur in childhood or adulthood. This type of trauma challenges the foundations of Cognitive Processing Therapy (CPT) because it intertwines various aspects of the human psyche—emotional, cognitive, and relational components all demand careful attention. The therapeutic journey for these individuals is seldom linear and requires clinicians to adapt and personalize their approach.

Complex trauma frequently results in what many describe as a disorder of identity. Survivors can struggle with a fragmented sense of self, as the trauma can disrupt normal development across emotional, relational, and cognitive domains. One of the main tasks in therapy is to help the client integrate these fragmented parts into a coherent sense of self, which can significantly influence therapy outcomes. A key factor in addressing this issue is fostering a therapeutic alliance that doesn't just aim to challenge distorted cognitions but also restores a sense of safety and identity.

Individuals with complex trauma often exhibit a range of symptoms beyond those typically seen in post-traumatic stress disorder (PTSD), including difficulties with emotional regulation, dissociation, and interpersonal relationships. For these clients, traditional CPT protocols may need adjustments to accommodate these broader symptom profiles without losing sight of the core therapeutic goals. This may involve integrating techniques from other therapeutic modalities, like Dialectical Behavioral Therapy (DBT), to enhance emotional regulation skills concurrently with cognitive restructuring techniques.

Establishing safety is always a preliminary goal in CPT, yet for those with complex trauma, this step becomes a prolonged and ongoing concern. Safety isn't merely about the absence of immediate crisis. It encompasses creating a therapeutic environment where clients feel emotionally secure enough to explore their trauma narratives and distorted beliefs. Therapists need to be adept at gauging the patient's readiness to confront trauma- related memories and beliefs, ensuring they maintain a balance between sufficient exposure and avoid retraumatization.

For survivors of complex trauma, dissociation can pose a unique challenge in CPT. Dissociative symptoms may range from mild forms, such as occasional zoning out, to more severe manifestations like dissociative identity disorder. Therapists need to be particularly mindful of these symptoms and may require training to recognize and work with dissociation. At times, pacing the therapy to allow time for grounding and reality orientation can improve engagement and reduce risk.

Given the complexity of the trauma, in some cases, it might be appropriate to extend the duration of CPT. Standard protocols might not be sufficient for clients with extensive trauma histories. An extended timeframe allows more room to build trust, to ensure the client's resources are cultivated adequately, and to address the different layers of trauma. It allows clients the latitude to revisit and revise their understanding of trauma with the guidance of their therapist.

The relational aspects of therapy are especially crucial for individuals with complex trauma. Their early interactions might have been marked by betrayal or abandonment, which can create profound mistrust in therapeutic settings. It's essential for therapists to demonstrate consistent empathy, reliability, and attuneness to their clients' needs. Establishing trustworthiness is an ongoing process that can significantly influence the trajectory and success of therapy.

Flexibility in therapeutic approaches is not simply advantageous but necessary when working with complex trauma. While CPT provides a structured approach, it's crucial that therapists remain adaptive to the evolving needs of their clients. It might be necessary to incorporate psychoeducation into the therapy to help clients understand their responses, normalize their experiences, and reduce shame associated with their symptomatology. Utilizing metaphors and analogies that resonate with the client's lived experiences can often bridge gaps in understanding and foster a deeper therapeutic engagement.

Additionally, working with complex trauma often necessitates collaboration with other professionals. Integrating insights from psychiatrists, social workers, and other therapists can strengthen the therapeutic process, ensuring that clients receive holistic and comprehensive care. Such collaboration also helps in addressing potential co-occurring disorders, such as depression or substance use issues, which are common among those with complex trauma histories.

Lastly, it's important for therapists themselves to remain aware of their own emotional and professional needs when working with complex trauma. The risk of vicarious trauma is heightened in these therapeutic relationships. Engaging in regular supervision, seeking peer support, and prioritizing self-care can help therapists maintain their well-being, ensuring they can offer the most effective care to their clients.

Complex trauma presents a distinct set of challenges and opportunities within CPT. By maintaining a flexible, empathic, and client-centered approach, therapists can effectively navigate the intricate landscape of trauma, facilitating meaningful transformation and healing for their clients.

CHAPTER 15

GROUP CPT SESSIONS

As we transition into the potential of group CPT sessions, we recognize an opportunity to cultivate a shared healing space that magnifies the individual therapeutic journey. Group therapy unfolds as a dynamic landscape where collective experiences offer new perspectives, validating personal narratives and reducing feelings of isolation often felt in trauma recovery.

Here, the structured framework of CPT, coupled with the supportive nature of groups, empowers participants through shared learning and communal resilience. The inherent benefits of group therapy, such as mutual encouragement and diversified insights, enrich the therapeutic alliance not only between therapist and patient but among group members themselves. By thoughtfully structuring sessions and being mindful of group dynamics, therapists can create an environment that is both safe and stimulating, inviting participants to explore and challenge maladaptive thought patterns in a collective setting. This approach not only fosters individual growth but establishes a community of healing, where shared victories and setbacks become stepping stones toward recovery.

Benefits of Group Therapy

In the realm of Cognitive Processing Therapy (CPT), group therapy sessions provide a unique and powerful platform for healing. While individual sessions offer personalized attention, group sessions create a sense of community and shared experience that can be transformative. When individuals come together to work through their traumas, it fosters an environment of mutual support and understanding. Participants can find solace in the fact that they are not alone in their struggles, which can often reduce feelings of isolation and alienation. This shared journey towards healing is one of the cornerstone benefits of group therapy.

Moreover, group therapy in the context of CPT allows individuals to observe the journey of others, providing both inspiration and a roadmap for their own progress. Witnessing peers confront their traumatic memories and maladaptive beliefs can motivate participants to tackle their challenges with renewed vigor and confidence. This atmosphere of collective courage can enhance personal growth that might take longer to achieve in individual therapy.

Another significant advantage of group therapy is the diversity of perspectives it brings. Each participant contributes a unique viewpoint shaped by their own experiences, beliefs, and insights. This diversity can lead to richer discussions and a deeper understanding of the cognitive patterns that trauma can engrain. Group members often learn new coping strategies and gain alternative perspectives that can illuminate blind spots in their understanding, helping them challenge and reframe their thoughts with greater efficacy.

Group therapy sessions also serve as a microcosm of larger social interactions, providing a safe space to practice new communication and interpersonal skills. Participants can experiment with expressing themselves and asserting their needs in a supportive environment, which can boost self-confidence and improve their relationships outside of therapy. This practice can be particularly beneficial for those whose trauma has impacted their ability to connect with others.

Empathy is another vital component fostered within group therapy. Listening to the stories of others and offering support in return helps participants develop a deeper sense of empathy—not only towards others but also for themselves. This self-compassion is a critical aspect of recovery as it allows individuals to forgive themselves and move forward without undue guilt or shame. Such emotional growth can significantly enhance the therapeutic outcomes of CPT.

Facilitators play a crucial role in harnessing the benefits of group therapy. Effective facilitators create a structured yet flexible environment where group members feel safe to explore and share their thoughts. They guide discussions to ensure that all voices are heard and that the group maintains its focus on therapeutic goals. By fostering a space of mutual respect and confidentiality, facilitators help build the trust necessary for deep healing work to occur.

The observational learning that occurs in group therapy should not be underestimated. As individuals witness others modeling healthy ways of thinking and behaving, they can internalize these patterns, integrating them into their own lives. This is an invaluable component of trauma recovery, where cognitive shifts are crucial. Group settings offer tangible, real-time examples of how Cognitive Processing Therapy principles can be applied effectively.

It's important to acknowledge the challenges of group therapy as well. For some, the idea of sharing personal traumas within a group can be daunting. It requires vulnerability and openness, which may not come easily for all. However, for those who choose to navigate this initial discomfort, the subsequent rewards often outweigh these challenges. As trust builds over time, many find that the group becomes a cornerstone of their healing journey.

Lastly, the cost-effectiveness of group therapy makes it an attractive option for many healthcare providers. Therapists can reach more individuals in a single session, which can be particularly advantageous in settings with resource constraints. This broader reach ensures that more people have access to healing interventions, potentially leading to greater overall community wellness.

In conclusion, the benefits of group therapy in Cognitive Processing Therapy are manifold. From fostering a sense of community and mutual support to enabling observational learning and diverse perspectives, group settings provide a fertile ground for profound therapeutic work. When guided by skilled facilitators, group therapy can lead to lasting transformations in participants' lives, paving the way for healing and empowerment.

Additionally, group therapy has been shown to enhance accountability and commitment to the therapeutic process. As participants share their progress and challenges with one another, there is a natural encouragement to stay engaged in treatment. This shared responsibility can increase motivation and foster a sense of belonging, as individuals see how their contributions impact others' journeys. Research has also demonstrated that people often experience faster recovery when they are part of a supportive group dynamic, as the collective effort can create a powerful momentum toward personal growth and healing.

Moreover, group therapy has the potential to normalize mental health struggles, reducing stigma and encouraging individuals to seek help earlier. As participants realize they are not alone in their experiences, they may feel more comfortable discussing sensitive issues openly. This shared vulnerability can promote emotional resilience and strengthen coping strategies, equipping participants with tools they can use long after therapy ends. In fact, studies have found that people who participate in group therapy are often more likely to continue practicing the skills they've learned, which can significantly enhance long-term outcomes.

Structuring Group Sessions

In the realm of Cognitive Processing Therapy (CPT), group sessions offer a unique opportunity to harness the collective wisdom and shared experiences of participants while promoting emotional healing and cognitive restructuring. Crafting a group session necessitates a delicate balance between structure and flexibility, allowing for a therapeutic environment where each member feels heard, valued, and understood.

The foundation of a well-structured group session lies in establishing clear objectives and expectations. From the outset, participants should understand the purpose of these gatherings: to provide support, challenge maladaptive thoughts, and foster personal growth. The therapist's role is to guide the group in a way that honors individual journeys while respecting collective goals. Each session becomes a tapestry of diverse thoughts woven together through guided discussions, exercises, and reflections.

At the beginning of a session, grounding techniques can be employed to create a sense of safety and readiness. A few moments of mindfulness or deep breathing can center the group, encouraging participants to transition from daily stressors to the therapeutic space. These initial moments are crucial for setting a tone of openness and calm, paving the way for deeper exploration and interaction.

A structured session often follows a predictable but adaptable pattern. Initiating with a brief check-in allows each participant to voice current emotions or challenges, fostering a sense of connection and empathy among group members. This check-in serves as a barometer for the group's emotional climate, guiding the therapist on where to focus efforts during that meeting.

Central to the session's progression are the primary activities or discussions that revolve around specific CPT concepts. These might include cognitive restructuring exercises, role-plays, or guided meditations centered on thought and emotional processing. Activities should be selected based on the group's specific needs and dynamics, ensuring they are relevant and engaging. In some groups, writing exercises may be introduced to streamline thoughts and encourage personal insights.

Facilitating group discussions can pose challenges, as therapists need to mediate varied perspectives while maintaining a therapeutic thread. Here, skillful questioning and empathetic listening become invaluable tools. While it's essential to encourage active participation, therapists must also be vigilant listeners, attuned to the nuances of what is said, and perhaps more importantly, what is not.

To maintain structure, time management becomes pivotal. Therapists should allocate time segments for each session component, allowing flexibility to delve deeper when the need arises. A rigorous adherence to the schedule can stifle spontaneity; thus, allowing organic discussions to flow within the agreed framework is beneficial.

As the session draws to a close, it's important to engage in a wrap-up process. Reflection activities or each member's summary of what they've learned help solidify the session's themes. This not only reinforces therapeutic progress but also anchors the day's work in collective memory. It prepares the group for applying insights outside the therapy room, a step essential in bridging therapy with everyday resilience.

Feedback mechanisms can offer critical insights for refining subsequent sessions. As part of structuring group therapy, therapists should regularly seek participant feedback to tailor approaches—increasing relevancy and improving engagement. Feedback also serves as an empowerment tool, validating participants' voices in the refinement of their therapeutic journey.

Finally, the ethos of confidentiality and mutual respect must be fiercely upheld throughout all sessions. Establishing and revisiting group norms at the beginning of each session can reinforce this foundation. Such norms not only safeguard individual privacy but also enhance trust within the group, laying the groundwork for effective collaborative work.

Ultimately, structuring group sessions in CPT is as much an art as it is a science, requiring a blend of clinical acumen, innovative thinking, and heartfelt empathy. When executed skillfully, these sessions become crucibles of change, where collective power transforms individual journeys into shared healing paths. By fostering an environment of insightful exploration and mutual support, group CPT sessions work towards the ultimate goal of reclaiming not just time and mental space, but a renewed sense of agency and community.

Incorporating regular participant feedback not only enhances the therapeutic process but also deepens participants' sense of ownership over their healing. Research has shown that when individuals feel they have a voice in shaping their treatment, they are more likely to stay engaged and actively participate. Feedback allows therapists to adjust their strategies, ensuring that each session is as relevant and impactful as possible. This adaptability is particularly valuable in group therapy settings, where diverse needs and backgrounds can result in varying levels of engagement and progress. By cultivating an open feedback loop, therapists can respond to emerging challenges and create a dynamic, responsive treatment environment that is more attuned to the group's evolving needs.

Furthermore, the importance of confidentiality and mutual respect cannot be overstated, as they are foundational to the success of group therapy. When individuals feel assured that their personal experiences will remain within the confines of the group, they are more likely to open up and engage in deeper, more meaningful conversations. This trust can significantly enhance the therapeutic outcomes of group Cognitive Processing Therapy, allowing participants to confront difficult emotions and experiences without fear of judgment or exposure. Studies have shown that groups with strong norms of confidentiality tend to experience higher levels of cohesion and therapeutic benefit, as members feel safe enough to share, process, and heal together. Thus, reinforcing these principles consistently ensures that the group remains a sanctuary of support and transformation.

Navigating Group Dynamics

In the realm of Group Cognitive Processing Therapy (CPT), understanding and navigating group dynamics is crucial for ensuring the success and therapeutic benefits of the sessions. The nature of group therapy introduces a layer of complexity that requires careful management of interpersonal interactions. Group dynamics can greatly influence the therapeutic process, and recognizing this is the first step towards managing them effectively.

At its core, group therapy functions as a microcosm of the outside world, reflecting social interactions in a controlled setting. Healthcare providers, therapists, and mental health professionals must first recognize that participants bring individual experiences, personalities, and copious underlying issues to the group. These can affect how one interacts with others and perceives the therapeutic process. For therapy to be effective, it's important to address and manage these varied dynamics actively.

One of the key elements in navigating group dynamics is fostering an environment of trust and safety. Members might initially feel exposed when sharing personal traumas and vulnerabilities. As facilitators, clinicians must cultivate an atmosphere that encourages openness and minimizes judgment. Protocols that establish respect and confidentiality within the group are non-negotiable. When members feel safe, they are more likely to engage wholly and benefit from shared experiences.

There is also a need to balance participation among group members. Every session includes diverse participants, each with their own pace and style of engagement. Some may monopolize conversations; others might struggle to speak up due to anxiety or shyness. It's essential to encourage those quieter members to share their thoughts, ensuring that each voice is heard. A balanced dynamic not only fosters inclusivity but also enriches the therapeutic process.

An effective technique for managing group dynamics is utilizing subgroups within the larger group. By creating smaller sets within the session, therapists can allow more intimate discussions, providing a platform for participants who might feel overwhelmed in larger settings. These smaller interactions can lead to deeper connections and promote a sense of belonging, which is often times pivotal for individuals dealing with PTSD.

As therapists guide these groups, maintaining a vigilant eye on the development of interpersonal dynamics is vital. There may arise conflicts or negative interactions that have the potential to derail the therapeutic process. Clinicians must be deft in addressing these issues, facilitating resolution and ensuring the focus remains on healing and growth. Participants, by observing how conflicts are navigated positively, can learn valuable interpersonal skills applicable beyond the therapy room.

Additionally, the diversity of experiences among participants offers a wealth of perspectives, fostering a learning environment. It's crucial that mental health professionals encourage participants to share their unique viewpoints and listen actively to others. Recognizing and valuing diverse experiences not only validates individual stories but also enhances collective understanding and empathy within the group.

Therapists must also remain aware of their own influence on group dynamics. Their demeanor, tone, and nonverbal cues can unconsciously set a tone for sessions. It's important that they model the communication and engagement they wish to see from participants. Consistent self- reflection and supervision can help therapists maintain this awareness and prevent their biases or stressors from influencing the group.

Another component of navigating group dynamics is education about generalized group behavior and what participants might experience. Preparing participants with knowledge of common reactions and emotions during group sessions can demystify the process and reduce anxiety. When individuals comprehend that fluctuations in emotions are normal and anticipated, they may be more open to fully engaging with the group.

Regular feedback sessions where group members can voice their thoughts on the dynamics and structure provide another layer of insight. Encouraging constructive feedback empowers participants and offers valuable data to therapists for adjusting strategies and handling dynamics more adeptly. Comments regarding what is effective and what isn't can direct both group and individual approaches in subsequent sessions.

In these collective healing spaces, it is critical to remind participants of the overarching goals of group CPT. While individual progress is important, the strength of group therapy lies in shared human experiences and support. This shared journey through trauma and healing creates bonds and mutual understanding that can foster post-treatment support networks among participants.

Ultimately, navigating group dynamics requires a blend of structure, empathy, and flexibility. Therapists must adapt their strategies as the group evolves, continually assessing and addressing the needs and dynamics of the members. This ongoing navigation is as much an art as it is a science—an ever-evolving dance that can lead to profound healing and transformation for those involved.

The success of a group CPT session doesn't just rest on individual achievements but also on the collective journey of the group. For healthcare providers and mental health professionals, the ability to expertly navigate these dynamics is a powerful tool in guiding participants from disparate backgrounds toward a common goal of healing and growth. Each session, while unique, offers an opportunity to reaffirm the importance of community, understanding, and resilience in the face of trauma.

CHAPTER 16

MANAGING THERAPIST CHALLENGES

As therapists navigate the complex landscape of guiding individuals through trauma recovery, they often face their own set of challenges that require careful attention and strategic management. It's vital to recognize that the therapist's emotional well-being is foundational not only to their professional effectiveness but also to their personal resilience. Avoiding burnout begins with setting clear boundaries and cultivating a robust support network, ensuring that practitioners are equipped with both the time and space to rejuvenate.

Addressing countertransference involves fostering self-awareness and mindfulness, which allow therapists to distinguish their own emotional responses from those of the client, fostering a therapeutic environment of empathy without over- identification. Supervision and peer support become lifelines in this process, offering fresh perspectives and shared experiences that can alleviate the sense of isolation and enhance professional growth. Managing these challenges is not about the absence of difficulty but rather involves embracing ongoing learning and self-care as integral components of a sustainable therapeutic practice.

Avoiding Burnout

As mental health professionals, the journey can be deeply rewarding yet profoundly challenging. The weight of our clients' trauma and suffering, combined with the demands of our personal lives, can lead to exhaustion. This exhaustion, if unchecked, can transform into burnout, a state of emotional, physical, and mental fatigue that saps our energy, creativity, and compassion. For therapists, who serve as pillars of support for clients, falling into burnout not only affects personal well-being but can also compromise the quality of care provided to those who depend on us.

Acknowledging and addressing the signs of burnout is the first step towards prevention. Symptoms can often manifest as physical tiredness, emotional detachment, reduced performance, and an increasing sense of helplessness or frustration. Early intervention is crucial, yet recognizing the issue within ourselves is sometimes the hardest step. Who cares for the caregiver? In truth, it must be the caregiver themselves. By cultivating

self-awareness and prioritizing self-care, therapists can create a buffer against the creeping shadow of burnout.

Often, burnout is not due to a single cause but a culmination of factors— high caseloads, emotionally taxing sessions, administrative duties, and even personal responsibilities. The nature of therapeutic work requires deep empathy and engagement, which can be draining when not balanced with restorative practices. Therefore, embedding a culture of self-care into our daily routines is indispensable. It's about finding the right balance, not just to survive in this field, but to thrive.

Creating clear boundaries between work and personal life is imperative. Make conscious efforts to disconnect from work after hours to recharge and rejuvenate. Even small actions, like setting specific times to check emails or limiting work-related calls outside working hours, can contribute to maintaining professional boundaries. Establishing these boundaries doesn't mean we care any less; it's about preserving our energy and passion for the long haul.

Cultivating a supportive network

also plays a vital role in combatting burnout. Connecting with peers for regular supervision or informal support groups can offer a safe space to share experiences and gain perspective. Colleagues, mentors, or professional networks provide emotional support and practical advice, which can alleviate feelings of isolation and stress.

Integrating mindfulness and relaxation techniques into daily routines can help maintain emotional balance. Mindfulness encourages staying present, managing stress, and gaining clarity—an antidote to the chaos that sometimes swirls in our professional lives. Consider incorporating practices such as meditation, deep breathing exercises, or yoga into your routine. These activities not only provide immediate relief but also promote long-term resilience.

Regularly reflecting on the impact of your work can also renew your sense of purpose and fulfillment. It's easy to get caught up in the minutiae of daily work and lose sight of the broader impact you have on your clients' lives. Take time to celebrate successes, however small they may seem. Reflecting on progress, witnessing clients' growth, and acknowledging your role in their healing journey can reignite your motivation and remind you of the vital contributions you make.

Engaging in continuous professional development can bolster your resilience against burnout. Learning new techniques and theories, attending workshops, or pursuing additional training can reinvigorate your practice. Staying informed about advancements in the field not only enhances your skills but also renews your passion and involvement in your career.

Don't underestimate the power of personal leisure activities and interests outside of therapy. Rediscover activities that bring joy, whether it's a creative hobby, outdoor activities, or spending quality time with loved ones. Cultivating a fulfilling life outside of work provides a nourishing counterbalance to professional demands, and helps prevent burnout by offering different sources of fulfillment and relaxation.

It's also essential to seek professional support when needed. Sometimes, connecting with a therapist or counselor who understands the unique pressures of our profession can be invaluable. They can offer objective insights, coping strategies, and the understanding needed to navigate the complexities of our experiences as therapists.

Ultimately, avoiding burnout is about sustaining oneself for the long journey. It's not a one-time fix but an ongoing commitment to recognizing personal limits, nurturing body and mind, and maintaining a supportive professional environment. By making strategic choices about workload, engaging in self-care, and fostering networks of support, therapists can continue to be effective, compassionate resources for their clients, while also nourishing their own well-being.

Therapists, as stewards of healing, must practice what they preach: self- care, ongoing reflection, and boundary-setting. Doing so not only protects our own health but ensures we remain effective, engaged, and empathetic providers for those we serve. Remember, we cannot draw from an empty well; replenishing our resources is a vital part of the work we do.

Dealing with Countertransference

In the realm of trauma therapy, countertransference isn't just a concept in a textbook; it's a lived experience that can deeply impact the therapeutic process. Therapists are not mere bystanders to their clients' stories. Instead, they're active participants who bring their own emotions, histories, and vulnerabilities into the therapeutic space. Understanding and navigating countertransference is crucial to maintaining the integrity of therapeutic work, especially when dealing with the complexities of trauma.

Countertransference, the emotional reactions and projections a therapist experiences towards a client, can subtly influence judgment and alter the therapist's objectivity. These reactions might include feelings of protectiveness, anger, or even inadequacy when faced with a client's distress. The first step in effectively managing countertransference is awareness. Therapists need to cultivate a strong sense of self-awareness and regularly engage in reflective practices to recognize their own emotional states.

Reflection, however, is just the beginning. Once a therapist has identified feelings of countertransference, it becomes essential to process these emotions constructively. Let's consider supervision, a cornerstone for managing these challenges. Supervision provides a supportive environment where therapists can discuss countertransference with experienced mentors. This shared experience offers fresh perspectives and strategies for managing emotional reactions, ensuring that these feelings do not obstruct the healing process.

While supervision is invaluable, therapists can also benefit from peer support groups where shared experiences create a sense of community. Within these groups, therapists can share experiences without fear of judgment, receiving feedback and insights from peers who understand the unique demands of trauma work. The sense of belonging can help diminish feelings of isolation and provide various strategies for dealing with challenging emotions.

But countertransference isn't merely an obstacle; it's a valuable tool in therapy. When managed properly, it offers insights into the therapeutic relationship and the client's world. For instance, if a therapist feels unexpectedly angry during a session, it may reflect unspoken anger within the client. Recognizing this can guide sensitive exploration, helping to identify and address underlying issues. Therefore, rather than ignoring these feelings, therapists should explore them to enhance the therapeutic alliance.

Another vital element in managing countertransference is self-care. The emotional weight carried by therapists working with trauma patients can be substantial. Engaging in regular self-care practices is not a luxury but a necessity to maintain emotional health. This could include activities that promote relaxation and rejuvenation—be it exercise, meditation, or hobbies that bring joy. By nurturing their own emotional well-being, therapists are better equipped to provide effective care to their clients.

Therapists should also strive to maintain clear boundaries with clients. Boundaries are fundamental to preventing countertransference from compromising professional judgment. By setting and adhering to these boundaries, therapists create a safe and ethical framework for therapy. Explicit boundaries help distinguish between the therapist's emotions and those of their clients, creating a more focused therapeutic process.

Mindfulness techniques can also play a pivotal role in managing emotional reactions. Techniques such as grounding exercises and deep breathing enable therapists to remain present, even when strong emotions arise. Being present helps in maintaining focus during sessions and allows therapists to respond thoughtfully rather than react impulsively to emotional cues.

Over time, therapists develop resilience as they learn to manage countertransference effectively. Each interaction becomes a learning opportunity, contributing to personal and professional growth. As therapists become more adept at recognizing and addressing their emotional responses, they enhance their ability to support their clients' healing journeys.

At its core, dealing with countertransference is about transformation— transforming impulsive reactions into reflective action, transforming emotional challenges into therapeutic insights, and ultimately, transforming both therapist and client through shared understanding and growth. This ongoing journey requires dedication to self-awareness, openness to support, and commitment to professional development. Embracing this process empowers therapists, allowing them to reclaim their mental space and provide the highest quality of care for those they serve.

Supervision and Support

Supervision and support are indispensable pillars for therapists, especially when navigating the challenges inherent in the world of trauma therapy. When dealing with complex cases, the insights and feedback from a more experienced colleague can be invaluable. Supervision not only provides a sounding board for therapists to discuss cases but also offers a critical space for personal and professional growth. In this setting, the therapist has the opportunity to reflect on their own reactions, biases, and emotional responses, which in turn enhances their capacity for empathy and understanding.

The landscape of supervision is diverse, and its form can vary significantly depending on the needs of the therapist and the setting in which they operate. One-on-one supervision is common, often involving regular meetings with a senior therapist. These sessions can include case discussions, role-playing, and the exploration of new therapeutic techniques. The supervisor's role is to offer guidance, help in identifying potential blind spots, and provide a safe space to discuss any discomforts or uncertainties. This dynamic relationship is built on trust and mutual respect, allowing the therapist to feel supported and validated in their journey.

Group supervision can be an enriching experience as well. Here, therapists gather to collaboratively discuss their cases, share insights, and learn from each other's experiences. This format fosters a sense of community and reduces feelings of isolation, which are common in the therapy profession. The diverse perspectives offered in a group setting can deepen understanding and spark innovative approaches to challenging cases. However, it requires skilled facilitation to ensure that each voice is heard and that discussions remain constructive and focused.

Beyond formal supervision, peer support networks play a crucial role in maintaining a therapist's well-being. Informal gatherings, whether in person or online, allow therapists to share experiences and advice in a more relaxed atmosphere. These networks can be particularly beneficial in reducing the sense of loneliness that can accompany work with high-trauma populations. As challenges are shared, therapists often find solidarity and encouragement among their peers, reinforcing their resilience and commitment to their work.

Self-care is another vital aspect interwoven with supervision and support. Therapists need to be attuned not only to the needs of their clients but also to their own. Regular supervision plays a preventative role against burnout by encouraging reflection on self-care practices. Discussing one's self-care habits with a supervisor or a peer can offer accountability and impetus to incorporate those practices diligently. It's a dual process where the focus is not only on improving therapeutic skills but also ensuring therapists remain mentally and emotionally vibrant.

Organizations can enhance the supervision and support for their therapists by cultivating a culture that prioritizes these elements. This includes offering regular training sessions, workshops focusing on coping skills, and providing resources to access personal therapy when needed. Leadership can play an active role by acknowledging the emotional toll of trauma work and creating policies that facilitate open dialogue and mutual support within the team. Flexible schedules, mental health days, and access to professional development resources are all means by which therapists can feel valued and supported.

It's important to acknowledge that supervision does not diminish the challenges therapists face but rather equips them with the necessary tools to tackle these challenges more effectively. As therapists progress in their careers, they might also step into the role of a supervisor themselves, embodying the dual role of learner and teacher. This transition carries its own set of challenges and requires a thoughtful approach to balance the demands of supporting others while continuing to seek personal guidance and learning.

In summary, robust supervision and support systems are essential for preventing burnout, enhancing therapeutic efficacy, and fostering the professional growth of therapists. As they face the emotional weight of their practice, these systems provide the scaffolding needed to navigate complex emotional landscapes effectively. By actively engaging in supervision and seeking support, therapists not only enrich their practice but also fortify their own mental well-being, ensuring they can continue to provide compassionate and competent care to their clients. In this manner, supervision and support underscore the interconnectedness of professional development and personal resilience, creating a sustainable path for long-term effectiveness in trauma therapy.

CHAPTER 17

OVERCOMING BARRIERS TO TREATMENT

In the journey to effectively treat PTSD, navigating barriers to treatment is essential for meaningful progress. These barriers, often deeply rooted in patient resistance, stigmatization, and a lack of motivation, can hinder even the most well-constructed therapeutic plans. Health care providers must approach these challenges with empathy, understanding the complex landscape of fears and misconceptions that patients carry. Encouraging open communication and fostering a safe, non-judgmental environment can help dissolve resistance and build trust.

It's crucial to address the stigma by normalizing therapy and validating the patient's experiences, removing the cloak of shame that often obscures their willingness to engage. Moreover, enhancing motivation isn't just about setting goals but aligning the therapeutic process with each individual's values and aspirations, thereby creating an intrinsic drive toward recovery. By empowering patients to take an active role in their healing journey, mental health professionals can make treatment not just a possibility, but a reality, one small step at a time.

One powerful way to normalize therapy and reduce stigma is through community engagement and education. Public awareness campaigns and outreach programs can help dispel myths surrounding mental health treatment, highlighting its benefits and promoting its accessibility. Studies indicate that when individuals see others from their own communities openly participating in therapy, they are more likely to seek help themselves. As therapy becomes a more accepted and celebrated part of wellness routines, it removes the barriers of shame that often prevent people from pursuing the care they need. This cultural shift can also contribute to greater societal support for mental health, ultimately creating a ripple effect that enhances the overall well-being of communities.

In addition, aligning therapy with personal values and aspirations has a profound impact on motivation and recovery. When individuals connect their therapeutic journey with their core beliefs—whether related to family, career, or personal growth—they are more likely to feel invested in the process. Research has shown that incorporating a client's intrinsic values into treatment plans can enhance their commitment and emotional investment, leading to more sustainable outcomes. This approach not only boosts engagement but also provides a deeper sense of purpose throughout recovery. By helping patients define their own path to healing, therapists can empower them to reclaim their autonomy and build resilience, fostering a sense of agency that makes each small step toward recovery feel both achievable and meaningful.

Patient Resistance

Engaging patients in therapy, particularly in the realm of Cognitive Processing Therapy (CPT) for PTSD, presents unique challenges. Among these, patient resistance is a significant barrier. It's a common thread that runs through clinical interactions, manifesting as a reluctance to delve into distressing memories or an aversion to therapeutic tasks. Understanding and addressing this resistance is crucial to facilitating meaningful progress in therapy.

Resistance often roots itself in the protective mechanisms developed by patients who've endured trauma. Over time, these individuals might have built robust defenses against revisiting painful experiences. These defenses, though maladaptive in the therapeutic context, have typically served as survival mechanisms outside it. To effectively address resistance, therapists need to approach it not as an adversary but as an intricate part of the healing process that calls for empathy and curiosity.

The therapeutic alliance plays a pivotal role in navigating resistance. Establishing trust and a sense of safety in the therapeutic space can soften resistance by creating an environment where patients feel seen and understood rather than judged. It's essential for therapists to foster an atmosphere where patients are invited to express their ambivalence or skepticism without fear of reprimand. Such openness can lead to breakthrough moments that propel therapy forward.

When addressing resistance, the language and approach of the therapist matter immensely. Empathetic communication that validates the patient's feelings and experiences can slowly unravel the reluctance to engage in therapy. Therapeutic inquiry should gently probe into the roots of resistance, helping the patient to explore the fears tied to change and vulnerability, which often underpin their resistance to treatment.

Implementing motivational interviewing techniques can also be beneficial. By aligning with the patient's own goals and values, therapists can encourage patients to articulate their reasons for change, weighing them against the cost of remaining entrenched in their current state. This empowerment-centric approach can help patients take ownership of their therapeutic journey.

It's also crucial to recognize that resistance might not always stem from conscious opposition. Sometimes, it arises from a deeper, subconscious level where the trauma is entrenched. This can manifest as forgetfulness, avoidance behavior, or cognitive dissonance, reflecting the internal conflict of wanting to heal while fearing the process. Addressing these layers requires patience and a willingness to move at a pace that respects the patient's readiness for change.

Cultural nuances add another layer of complexity to patient resistance. Diverse backgrounds and belief systems can influence how trauma is perceived and how patients engage with therapy. Hence, cultural competence and sensitivity are indispensable. Recognizing and respecting cultural values aids in lessening resistance and enhancing engagement.

Therapists should also be acutely aware of their own responses to patient resistance. It's a natural instinct to feel frustrated when progress seems stalled, yet it's imperative to remain supportive and avoid interpreting resistance as a personal affront or a failure in therapeutic technique. Instead, it's an invitation to delve deeper, adapt strategies, and innovate within the therapeutic framework.

Collaboration is another key strategy in managing resistance. Engaging patients as active participants in their treatment planning not only empowers them but also allows for therapy to be more tailored to their specific needs and concerns. When patients contribute to setting their therapeutic goals and are involved in monitoring their progress, they are more likely to feel invested in the process.

Furthermore, keeping an open dialogue about what might be contributing to their resistance can be incredibly useful. Questions that explore what patients find challenging about therapy or what they feel could improve their experience can provide important insights and opportunities for therapeutic adjustments that reduce barriers to engagement.

Patient resistance is an inherent part of the therapeutic process that offers significant learning opportunities for both the patient and the therapist. By approaching resistance with compassion, curiosity, and cultural understanding, therapists can transform this barrier into a bridge that leads to deeper understanding and healing. The journey through resistance may be complex, but it is peppered with invaluable insights and the potential for genuine, lasting change.

Resistance in therapy often reflects underlying fears, past trauma, or deep-seated beliefs that need careful exploration and understanding. Rather than viewing resistance as a roadblock, many therapists embrace it as a sign of active engagement with the therapeutic process. Research has shown that when resistance is met with empathy and open-ended questions, it can lead to breakthroughs in understanding and new perspectives. By acknowledging the patient's internal struggles, therapists can create a safe space where these feelings can be unpacked and addressed. This process not only allows patients to work through their barriers but also encourages self-awareness and emotional growth, making it a crucial part of the healing journey.

Cultural competence plays a critical role in navigating resistance effectively. Each patient brings their own set of cultural values, beliefs, and life experiences to therapy, which may influence how they perceive and react to treatment. For example, some individuals may view seeking therapy as a sign of weakness due to societal or familial expectations, while others may feel a deep mistrust of the mental health system based on historical experiences within their communities. Therapists who approach resistance with cultural humility and sensitivity can better understand these unique challenges and tailor their interventions accordingly. Studies show that when therapists demonstrate cultural understanding, patients are more likely to engage fully in the therapeutic process, allowing for a deeper and more productive exploration of resistance and ultimately fostering long-term healing.

Addressing Stigmatization

Stigmatization surrounding mental health and PTSD, in particular, remains a formidable barrier to treatment. It's a multifaceted issue that impacts not only the individual seeking help but also shapes the broader perceptions of communities and healthcare systems. The key to addressing stigmatization in the context of PTSD is to understand the roots of stigma, its manifestations, and the strategic pathways we can adopt to dismantle its lasting influence.

At its core, stigma is nurtured by misinformation and fear. When individuals are unaware of the realities of PTSD, misconceptions flourish, leading to unfair judgments. For healthcare providers and mental health professionals, a pivotal step in dismantling stigma is education. Educators at all levels must provide accurate, comprehensive information about PTSD, clarifying myths and highlighting facts. This can reshape both public perceptions and organizational policies, creating a ripple effect that makes seeking help more acceptable and accessible.

The impact of stigma can manifest in numerous ways. Patients may fear being labeled as "mentally unstable" or "weak," concerns that arise both in personal and professional settings. This fear of judgment can deter individuals from seeking treatment altogether. For mental health professionals, it is paramount to cultivate a supportive environment that encourages openness and acceptance. By openly discussing the potential for stigma in initial sessions, therapists can work to validate their patients' concerns and foster a sense of safety.

Addressing stigmatization requires deliberate strategies beyond simple education. Advocacy plays an essential role—both within communities and larger policy-making spheres. Healthcare providers have the unique opportunity to leverage their authority and expertise to advocate for systemic change. This means pushing for mental health to be prioritized in healthcare agendas and ensuring that insurance policies and workplace norms reflect an understanding and respect for mental health challenges.

Furthermore, integrating cultural competence in treatment approaches can help mitigate stigma, particularly in diverse populations. Cultural nuances significantly influence how mental health is perceived and treated. Mental health professionals need to be sensitive to these differences and tailor their interventions accordingly, recognizing that stigma may have deep- rooted cultural undertones.

One effective way to address stigma within therapy sessions is through language. The words we choose can either reinforce or dismantle stereotypes and misconceptions. Using person-first language, such as "individual experiencing PTSD" instead of "PTSD sufferer," emphasizes that a diagnosis does not define the person. Language should be empowering rather than labeling, encouraging patients to see themselves beyond their trauma.

In addition to these strategies, storytelling emerges as a powerful tool in combating stigma. Sharing stories of recovery and resilience can humanize the experience of PTSD, offering hope and connection. These narratives can be shared through group therapy sessions, public forums, or media platforms. For patients, hearing and sharing stories helps normalize their experiences and build a supportive community.

Mental health professionals can also harness the potential of technology to combat stigma. Social media campaigns, online educational resources, and virtual support groups can expand the reach of anti-stigma messages. By leveraging digital tools, we can connect with a broader audience, fostering a wider understanding and acceptance of PTSD and its treatment.

Finally, involving former patients as advocates or peer supporters can significantly reduce stigma. Those who have journeyed through PTSD treatment bring invaluable perspective and credibility. Their involvement can help bridge gaps between patients and providers, offering lived experiences as testimony to the reality and manageability of living with PTSD.

Ultimately, the journey to eradicate stigmatization is continuous and requires collective effort. By combining education, advocacy, language, and technology, mental health professionals can build a foundation of understanding that supports individuals in seeking and benefitting from treatment. In doing so, we move closer to a world where mental health is embraced with the empathy and respect it deserves, allowing every individual the dignity of receiving care without prejudice or fear.

Technology offers an unprecedented opportunity to reach diverse and far-flung populations, breaking down the geographical and social barriers that often inhibit access to mental health resources. Virtual platforms such as webinars, online workshops, and mental health podcasts can play a vital role in normalizing discussions around PTSD, making information more accessible to a global audience. Additionally, online communities and forums allow individuals to share their experiences, find solidarity, and receive emotional support without fear of judgment. Studies have shown that digital mental health resources can significantly reduce the stigma associated with seeking help, as they provide a sense of anonymity and comfort for those who might otherwise avoid face-to-face interactions. By capitalizing on these tools, mental health professionals can help change the narrative surrounding PTSD, emphasizing healing and resilience over shame and isolation.

Involving former patients as advocates or peer supporters can serve as a powerful tool in transforming societal perceptions of PTSD. These individuals bring credibility, authenticity, and a unique perspective that can deeply resonate with others who are struggling. Peer support not only validates the experiences of current patients but also promotes hope and motivation by demonstrating that recovery is possible. Research shows that peer-led initiatives can increase engagement in treatment, reduce feelings of alienation, and encourage individuals to seek care earlier in their recovery process. Furthermore, when individuals see others who have faced similar challenges successfully managing their PTSD, it can significantly diminish the fear and stigma associated with mental health treatment. This approach creates a supportive, empathetic environment where patients feel understood and empowered, ultimately contributing to a shift in the broader cultural attitudes towards mental health.

Enhancing Motivation

One of the most significant barriers to treatment in Cognitive Processing Therapy (CPT) is ensuring that patients remain engaged and motivated. Without motivation, the therapeutic process can stall or even regress, making it essential to address this aspect head-on. Motivation can wane for various reasons, including experiencing overwhelming emotions, confronting challenging beliefs, or feeling disconnected from the therapeutic goals. It's crucial for therapists to recognize and understand these deterrents to reignite the patient's drive toward recovery.

To foster motivation, the first step is creating an empathetic and understanding therapeutic environment. Patients need to feel valued and understood, which starts with active listening. When a therapist fully listens, patients feel supported, which can reignite their willingness to engage. This foundational understanding helps foster a sense of safety where patients can explore their thoughts and emotions without fear of judgment, making them more likely to invest in the therapy process.

Additionally, setting realistic and achievable goals is necessary for motivation. Goals should align with the patient's values and desires, creating a sense of ownership and personal relevance. By breaking down overarching objectives into smaller, manageable tasks, patients can celebrate incremental successes. Each achievement propels the patient forward, boosting their motivation. Therapists might employ motivational interviewing techniques to help patients articulate their goals and discover the intrinsic motivations underlying their journey toward healing.

Acknowledging and addressing ambivalence is another strategy. Ambivalence towards change is natural, especially for patients confronting deep-seated trauma. Therapists who skillfully navigate this ambivalence can help patients verbalize their conflicting feelings, allowing them to explore the pros and cons of change in a supportive setting. This dialogue often leads to patients discovering personal motivations for change they may not have previously recognized.

The therapeutic alliance plays a crucial role in maintaining motivation. Establishing and sustaining a strong bond between therapist and patient creates a collaborative space where patients feel respected and empowered. When patients trust their therapist, they are more inclined to remain open about their struggles and successes, keeping the lines of communication active. Strong rapport not only motivates patients but can also rejuvenate therapists, fueling their own passion and dedication to the work.

Incorporating psychoeducation into sessions can heighten motivation by increasing patients' understanding of PTSD and its effects. When patients comprehend more about their condition and recognize that their symptoms and reactions are part of a normal response to trauma, they often feel a renewed sense of hope. This knowledge dispels myths and stigmatizing beliefs, replacing them with evidence-based truths that encourage patient engagement.

Motivation can also be enhanced through cognitive restructuring, where patients learn to identify and challenge maladaptive thoughts that hinder their progress. By replacing these thoughts with positive, affirming beliefs, patients not only change their perception of past events but also their approach to therapy. This shift can light a motivational spark that encourages ongoing participation in the therapeutic process.

Empowering patients is vital. When patients are given tools and strategies to help them manage their own progress, they often feel a greater sense of control and motivation. Techniques like mindfulness, self-reflection, and self-compassion practices can be incredibly empowering. When patients notice their ability to influence their emotional and cognitive experiences, their investment in therapy usually increases.

It's essential to remain adaptable and attentive to a patient's evolving needs. Therapy isn't a one-size-fits-all process, and what motivates one patient might not work for another. Regularly checking in with patients about their therapy experience can provide valuable insights and allow for the adaptation of strategies to maintain motivation over time.

Ultimately, enhancing motivation is about creating a partnership built on trust, empathy, and empowerment. It's about recognizing each patient's unique journey and facilitating a space where they feel motivated to explore, challenge, and heal. As therapists and mental health professionals, the goal is to work alongside our patients, not just as guides, but as collaborators in the shared mission of reclaiming mental space and well-being.

Incorporating personalized strategies into therapy can also enhance long-term motivation by aligning treatment with each patient's strengths, preferences, and values. For instance, some patients may respond well to goal-setting techniques, while others might find meaning in creative expression through art or journaling. Research supports the idea that when therapy is tailored to fit the individual's preferred coping mechanisms and personal interests, it can result in greater engagement and more meaningful progress. Additionally, involving patients in decision-making processes—such as choosing therapeutic exercises or setting session goals—can foster a sense of ownership and autonomy over their healing journey.

This participatory approach not only boosts self-efficacy but also strengthens the therapeutic alliance, which has been shown to be one of the most significant predictors of successful treatment outcomes.

Furthermore, maintaining motivation throughout therapy is often linked to the establishment of achievable milestones that celebrate incremental progress. Celebrating small victories—whether it's managing a difficult emotion or successfully applying a coping strategy in real life—helps patients feel a sense of accomplishment and forward momentum. Studies have found that recognizing these small wins can reduce feelings of helplessness and increase self-esteem, reinforcing a patient's belief in their ability to manage their mental health. This approach fosters a sense of continuity and growth, reminding patients that every step, no matter how small, contributes to their overall healing. By remaining adaptable and consistently validating progress, therapists can help patients stay motivated throughout the sometimes challenging path to recovery.

CHAPTER 18

EVALUATING PROGRESS IN THERAPY

Assessing progress in therapy is essential for both the client and the practitioner, providing pivotal insights into the effectiveness of the treatment and guiding necessary adjustments. As therapists, the journey of monitoring patient change is as crucial as initiating therapy itself, demanding a compassionate yet structured approach.

Regular evaluations allow us to gauge the individual's evolution, honoring their unique healing process while ensuring that they are not only moving forward but doing so at a comfortable pace. We must be vigilant in recognizing when it's time to shift or refine the treatment strategy, fueled by continuous feedback and collaborative dialogue with our clients. This dynamic interplay of monitoring and modifying treatment plans not only enhances the therapeutic alliance but also empowers clients to reclaim autonomy over their healing journey. Let's stay committed to adjusting our lenses, striking a balance between clinical acumen and empathy, as we guide our clients towards reclaiming their mental space with resilience and hope.

One of the most effective ways to assess progress is through regular, structured check-ins that allow clients to reflect on their own experiences. By asking open-ended questions that encourage introspection, therapists can uncover subtle shifts in the client's mindset or behavior that may not be immediately apparent. Research has shown that clients who engage in self-reflection during therapy tend to develop deeper insights and feel more involved in the process. These moments of reflection provide valuable opportunities for both the client and therapist to track progress, celebrate achievements, and identify areas that may require further exploration. This collaborative approach helps maintain momentum, as clients begin to see how their thoughts, feelings, and actions are changing over time, reinforcing their sense of agency in the therapeutic process.

Measuring progress can be enriched by incorporating a variety of assessment tools, including standardized questionnaires, self-report measures, and behavioral tracking. These tools provide concrete data that can offer both the therapist and client a clearer picture of progress. For instance, using a symptom-tracking tool in conjunction with subjective feedback allows for a more holistic view of treatment outcomes. This dual approach—qualitative and quantitative—helps therapists make informed decisions about the direction of therapy, ensuring that adjustments are not only timely but also based on a thorough understanding of the client's evolving needs. Studies have shown that a combination of objective measures and client self-report can improve treatment outcomes, as it offers a comprehensive approach to progress evaluation.

It's also essential to recognize that progress is not always linear, and setbacks may occur along the way. In fact, research on therapeutic change indicates that periods of stagnation or even regression can be a natural part of the healing process, particularly in complex conditions like PTSD or anxiety. These moments can provide valuable opportunities for therapists to revisit the client's coping strategies and reframe challenges as part of the learning process. By embracing setbacks with compassion and curiosity, therapists can help clients reframe these moments not as failures but as temporary obstacles that can be overcome with continued effort and support. This shift in perspective can bolster resilience and provide a sense of hope, reminding clients that healing is often an iterative, evolving journey.

Lastly, progress assessment should always be accompanied by an emphasis on the therapeutic relationship itself. Strong therapeutic alliances have been consistently linked with better outcomes, and the process of assessing progress can reinforce this bond. Regular, open communication about treatment goals, progress, and potential challenges fosters trust, transparency, and collaboration between therapist and client. Clients are more likely to engage fully in the therapeutic process when they feel their therapist is genuinely invested in their progress, responsive to their needs, and adaptable to their changing circumstances. In this way, progress assessments not only help track clinical improvements but also deepen the connection between therapist and client, creating a supportive environment in which healing can truly thrive.

Monitoring Patient Change

In therapy, particularly in cognitive processing therapy (CPT) for post- traumatic stress disorder (PTSD), monitoring patient change is not just a methodological requirement but a reflection of the transformative journey undertaken by the patient. Notably, tracking progress is fundamental to the therapeutic process as it offers both the therapist and patient a lens through which to understand shifts in cognition, emotion, and behavior. The nature of PTSD means that changes can be incremental but profound, unfolding in complex ways that require a nuanced view.

Every step in the patient's journey is significant. Progress isn't always linear; it may slow, plateau, or even regress at times, which can be discouraging without proper guidance. For health care providers, keeping an empathetic and motivational tone can help sustain the patient's momentum. Therapists are encouraged to foster an environment where patients feel their small victories are celebrated and setbacks are framed as opportunities for growth rather than failures.

The first measure of patient change involves observable shifts in how patients narrate their trauma. Revisiting their trauma accounts can illustrate progress in how they process and articulate their experiences. An initial narrative might be fragmented and emotionally charged, but over time, with ongoing therapy, the narrative often becomes more coherent and less distress-laden. This shift is crucial, as it demonstrates a modicum of mastery over a narrative that once overwhelmed them.

In addition, therapists should pay close attention to changes in thought patterns and beliefs. Cognitive distortions, such as overgeneralization or catastrophizing, tend to soften as patients progress. The use of cognitive restructuring techniques supports this transformation by helping patients challenge and revise these maladaptive thoughts. Regularly revisiting thought records can provide both therapist and patient with tangible evidence of change, reinforcing self-efficacy and the therapeutic alliance.

While cognitive shifts are crucial, monitoring emotional progress is equally important. Patients often learn to recognize and name their emotions more accurately as therapy continues. Strategies for managing intense emotions become part of their repertoire, enabling a healthier interaction with their emotional landscape. The change can be seen in their ability to engage with feelings of anger, sadness, or fear without becoming overwhelmed.

In addition, part of monitoring change is taking note of how patients adjust to and manage their daily lives. The impact of PTSD on everyday functioning is profound; thus, seeing patients engage more fully with their life—such as maintaining relationships, returning to work, or resuming hobbies—are critical indicators of improvement. This kind of progress should be documented and discussed in sessions to affirm patients' advancements and encourage continued growth.

Therapists must also consider patient feedback. Direct feedback offers invaluable insights that can inform the direction of therapy and ensure that it remains aligned with patient needs. Encouraging open communication about what strategies are working well or which areas feel neglected can refine the treatment process and make it more patient-centered and effective.

Utilizing standardized assessment tools is another practice to measure patient change systematically. Questionnaires and symptom tracking tools can provide a quantitative analysis of progress, highlighting variations in symptom intensity and frequency. While not a substitute for the qualitative insights gained through observation and conversation, these tools offer another dimension to understanding change that can help shape ongoing treatment planning.

Adjusting treatment plans based on progress is a skill that all therapists should cultivate. As patients evolve, their needs in therapy may change. This requires flexibility and a willingness to adapt approaches without deviating from the overall goals. Therapists might introduce new interventions, increase focus on certain aspects of therapy, or even slow down the pace if necessary, all tailored to sustain and enhance therapeutic outcomes.

Despite careful monitoring, unexpected challenges can arise, requiring immediate attention and recalibration of the treatment approach. Patience and resilience, both from the therapist and patient, are essential here. By framing challenges as a natural part of the healing process, therapists can mitigate the frustration or hopelessness a patient might feel when adversity strikes.

Fundamentally, successful monitoring of patient change in therapy for PTSD is not merely about measuring symptom reduction. It encapsulates a broader narrative of recovery, depicting a person's journey towards reclaiming their agency, resilience, and a renewed capacity for hope and connection. By thoroughly understanding and recording this process, healthcare professionals can better support each patient's uniqueness, advocating for their nuanced needs while providing a launchpad for enduring healing.

Adjusting Treatment Plans

As we explore the journey of evaluating progress in therapy, the ability to adjust treatment plans dynamically emerges as a cornerstone in the provision of effective care. Each client we encounter brings with them a unique tapestry of experiences, challenges, and resiliencies. Our therapeutic task, therefore, is not to fit them into a rigid framework but to allow the framework of the Cognitive Processing Therapy (CPT) to bend and shift to accommodate their individual needs. This adaptability is not merely beneficial but essential for fostering genuine healing.

Adjusting a treatment plan begins with recognizing the fluid nature of both trauma and healing. Symptoms of Post-Traumatic Stress Disorder (PTSD) and related maladaptive thoughts are not static; they can ebb and flow in unexpected ways. As clinicians, we must be vigilant and perceptive to these fluctuations. This means regularly assessing both the verbal and non-verbal cues of our clients, adopting a mindset of continuous evaluation, and being prepared to pivot strategies at various stages of the therapeutic process.

Crucially, treatment adjustments should be rooted in collaborative dialogue. Engaging clients actively in discussions about their goals and progress fosters a sense of ownership and empowerment. This collaborative approach furthers their autonomy and affirms their role as partners in the healing process.

By encouraging an open exchange, we can gather insights that might otherwise remain hidden, such as subtle shifts in mood or emergent stressors outside the therapy room.

Empathy and flexibility are indispensable in this process. Consider a client who initially struggles with the practice of writing a trauma narrative. Should we insist on this method rigidly, we might inadvertently reinforce a sense of distress or helplessness. Instead, we can adapt the approach by perhaps incorporating verbal storytelling or using creative expressions like art or music, aligning more closely with the client's comfort zone. By tailoring the process, we not only reduce potential harm but also draw nearer to the client's authentic self-expression.

Therapists should also be attuned to the potential for modality fatigue. Consistent engagement with CPT tasks can sometimes lead clients to feel overwhelmed or disheartened. At such junctures, a return to the basics of emotional regulation strategies or a pause for reflection and consolidation of learning may be appropriate. These adjustments serve as a reminder that therapy is not a linear trajectory but an adaptable journey that respects the natural rhythm of healing.

In some scenarios, adjusting treatment plans involves integrating additional therapeutic techniques. For instance, a client showing resilience but still struggling with particular belief systems might benefit from incorporating mindfulness practices alongside cognitive restructuring. Similarly, clients experiencing co-occurring disorders may require the incorporation of interventions tailored to address specific symptoms of those conditions. Such integrations should be evidence-based and thoughtfully aligned with the core tenets of CPT, ensuring coherence and reinforcing the primary therapeutic objectives.

Feedback mechanisms play a pivotal role in guiding these adjustments. Utilizing structured feedback tools or more informal check-ins can richly inform our understanding of a client's progress and hurdles. Gathering feedback is not merely about addressing shortcomings but celebrating achievements. Recognizing and affirming small victories bolsters motivation and can ignite a renewed commitment to the therapeutic process.

Moreover, clinicians should remain mindful of the cultural context and societal factors that may influence treatment outcomes. Cultural competence is critical when considering adjustments to treatment plans. A nuanced understanding of cultural background, language preferences, and social determinants of health can guide tailored interventions that respect and honor the diversity of clients' lived experiences. This may mean modifying traditional therapeutic techniques to better align with cultural norms or values.

Ultimately, the ability to modify treatment plans requires that therapists hold a space of humility and curiosity. It involves acknowledging that while we bring expertise in therapy, the client's lived experience is the ultimate guide. Our role is to constantly refine our approach based on the evolving narrative of the client's journey. This approach demands ongoing professional development and a commitment to lifelong learning, ensuring that we remain adaptive and responsive to emerging therapeutic insights.

In conclusion, adjusting treatment plans in therapy is an art that combines attentive observation, theoretical knowledge, and empathetic engagement. It requires courage to stray from a set plan and intuition to identify when change is necessary. As clinical supervisors, researchers, and therapists, embracing this adaptability not only enriches our professional practice but most importantly, paves the way for genuine transformation in the lives of those we serve. Through fostering a responsive and client- centered therapeutic environment, we take meaningful strides towards empowerment and healing, delivering on the promise that therapy offers to reclaim mental space and foster well-being.

Utilizing Feedback

In the realm of trauma therapy, particularly within the scope of Cognitive Processing Therapy (CPT), feedback is not merely a tool—it's a cornerstone of therapeutic progress. Incorporating feedback effectively can transform the therapeutic process, making it more tailored and responsive to each patient's unique needs. The dynamic use of feedback fosters a collaborative environment where both therapist and patient engage in an ongoing dialogue, continuously shaping the course of therapy.

Feedback serves multiple purposes in therapy. It can validate the patient's experiences, highlight areas of significant progress, and identify challenges that need more attention. In applying feedback, therapists encourage patients to reflect on their patterns of thought and behavior. This reflection, in turn, empowers the patient to become an active participant in their healing process. The inclusion of patient feedback allows for adjustments in therapeutic techniques and strategies, tailoring interventions to better suit the patient's evolving needs.

The process of gathering feedback should be structured yet flexible. Regular check-ins, whether at the beginning or end of sessions, can facilitate an open line of communication. These moments create a safe space for the patient to express their thoughts on what is working and what isn't. Questions should be open-ended, allowing for rich, qualitative insights. For instance, asking a patient how they felt after trying a specific cognitive restructuring technique can yield valuable information that purely quantitative measures might miss.

From a therapist's perspective, evaluating feedback requires an empathetic and non-defensive approach. It's important to remember that feedback is not personal criticism but a vital tool for refining therapeutic methods.

Constructive feedback helps in refining approaches and ensuring they align with the therapeutic goals initially set. Therapists should welcome feedback with gratitude and openness, even when it challenges their current approach. It's a chance to grow and fine-tune the therapeutic journey.

An important concept when utilizing feedback is the idea of adjusting treatment plans. Feedback may reveal that certain strategies are not as effective as anticipated. Flexibility is crucial here, allowing therapists to modify their approach in real time. This might mean shifting focus to another intervention, trying a different CPT technique, or even revisiting and revising therapy goals to better align with the patient's current context and capabilities.

Mental health professionals should be prepared to guide patients in giving specific and actionable feedback. It's not uncommon for patients to initially struggle with articulating their thoughts on therapy. Providing examples and encouraging descriptive feedback can bridge this gap. For example, rather than a vague "it didn't work," guiding patients towards specifics like "I struggled to challenge my thought because it feels ingrained" provides more useful information. This specificity aids in developing targeted interventions that address particular barriers or concerns.

Incorporating feedback also requires a consideration of cultural and personal context. Different patients may have unique perceptions of mental health and therapy based on their backgrounds, and these perceptions will inevitably influence the feedback they provide. Therapists must be culturally sensitive and aware, adapting their interpretations of feedback accordingly and checking in with patients to validate these understandings. Feedback isn't just about what happens during sessions— it's also influenced by what happens outside therapy and in the patient's real world. Recognizing this broader context is critical to effective therapy.

Beyond patient feedback, therapists should also actively seek feedback from peers and supervisors. Peer supervision and group consultations are invaluable resources for gaining additional perspectives on therapeutic approaches. Regular peer reviews and discussions can provide insights that might not be apparent in individual practice and can help address any blind spots in therapy. It also ensures therapists remain accountable and grounded in the best practices and ethical standards of CPT.

Finally, the efficacy of feedback in CPT relies heavily on the established therapeutic alliance. Without a strong foundation of trust and openness, feedback can feel intimidating or even counterproductive. Therapists must work to create and maintain an environment where patients feel safe sharing their honest experiences and observations. This safety is cultivated through consistent active listening, empathy, and mutual respect, reinforcing the belief that the therapeutic space is one of understanding and growth.

In closing, utilizing feedback in therapy is not a static task but a dynamic process. It requires continuous engagement, adaptation, and an unwavering commitment to personalizing the healing journey. As therapists integrate feedback thoughtfully, they not only enhance the therapeutic process but also empower patients to reclaim control over their healing, encouraging resilience and autonomy in the face of trauma.

CHAPTER 19

INTEGRATING TECHNOLOGY IN CPT

As we advance into an increasingly digital world, integrating technology into Cognitive Processing Therapy (CPT) brings a wealth of opportunities to enhance therapeutic outcomes. Digital tools can provide a flexible and accessible platform that complements traditional therapy methods, helping to bridge gaps between sessions and engage patients more dynamically. Teletherapy, particularly, ensures individuals can access support regardless of geographical or physical limitations, thereby removing barriers to consistent treatment. It's essential to remain mindful of ethical considerations, ensuring patient confidentiality and data security are maintained.

By thoughtfully incorporating technological advancements, mental health professionals can foster a more responsive and inclusive therapeutic environment, ultimately helping individuals reclaim their time and mental space to lead lives less burdened by the shadows of trauma. This chapter invites readers to embrace these innovations with both enthusiasm and caution, ensuring an ethical and empathetic approach to digital CPT practices.

As technology continues to evolve, its potential to enhance therapeutic practices becomes increasingly apparent. Digital Cognitive Processing Therapy (CPT) tools, such as mobile apps, virtual reality simulations, and online support groups, offer opportunities for patients to engage with therapeutic content in ways that align with their individual needs and schedules. For instance, virtual reality (VR) has shown promise in treating PTSD by immersing patients in controlled environments where they can confront and process traumatic memories in a safe, structured manner. Studies indicate that VR-based therapies can help patients reduce the intensity of trauma-related flashbacks, anxiety, and avoidance behaviors. When integrated with traditional therapeutic modalities, these tools not only expand the reach of CPT but also enhance the ability to tailor treatment to each patient's specific challenges and preferences.

However, it is crucial to approach the integration of technology into therapy with caution to maintain the quality and integrity of care. While digital tools offer convenience and accessibility, they also present challenges such as ensuring adequate user engagement, maintaining a strong therapeutic alliance, and addressing the potential for technological dependence. Mental health professionals must carefully consider how technology is used within the context of treatment, ensuring it enhances rather than diminishes the therapeutic relationship. Research shows that technology can be most effective when it supplements, rather than replaces, in-person interactions, allowing for the continuity of human connection that is essential for trust and healing. By embracing a balanced approach that incorporates both the innovations of digital tools and the foundational principles of compassionate, personalized care, therapists can create a more responsive and inclusive environment for healing.

Use of Digital Tools

As we forge ahead in modern therapy, digital tools have become indispensable in bridging gaps and elevating the quality of care provided in Cognitive Processing Therapy (CPT). Digital platforms and applications serve not only as a source of information but also as interactive aids that empower both therapists and clients. These tools create a space for continuous engagement, allowing individuals to work on their healing journey even outside the confines of traditional therapy sessions. This shift harnesses technology to cater to the contemporary needs of mental health professionals, enhancing the efficiency and accessibility of CPT.

For therapists navigating the complexities of PTSD treatment, digital tools offer an array of benefits. They provide real-time data collection and analysis, facilitating a deeper understanding of the client's progress and challenges. With the aid of apps and software, therapists can monitor homework completion, track mood changes, and receive insights into clients' thought patterns between sessions. This data-driven approach allows for more personalized and dynamic treatment plans, ensuring that interventions are precisely targeted to the individual's needs.

Moreover, online platforms offer a repository of resources that can be accessed by clients anytime, fostering a sense of independence and self- efficacy. Clients can engage with educational materials, practice exercises, and complete assignments on their own schedule. This kind of flexibility is crucial for those who may find strict appointment schedules

challenging due to work, family commitments, or other barriers. Access to therapy resources in a digital format empowers clients to take an active role in their healing, making the therapeutic process collaborative and client-centric.

Digital tools also enhance the therapist-client relationship by promoting consistent communication and support. Secure messaging systems integrated into therapy apps allow for ongoing dialogue, providing clients with the reassurance that help is always available when needed.

These platforms enable therapists to offer timely feedback, keep track of client concerns, and adjust therapeutic strategies quickly as situations evolve. This immediacy in communication strengthens the therapeutic alliance, encouraging transparency and mutual trust.

Additionally, virtual reality (VR) technology is emerging as a promising tool in the therapeutic landscape. VR offers controlled environments where clients can safely confront and process traumatic events under the guidance of a therapist. This immersive experience can be tailored to individual needs, helping clients gradually desensitize and reframe their understanding of traumatic memories. While still in its infancy, VR holds potential for profound therapeutic breakthroughs as more therapists incorporate it into their practice.

Privacy and security remain paramount when integrating technology into CPT. It's essential that therapists and clinics employ platforms that comply with HIPAA regulations to ensure the confidentiality of client information. As more personal data is collected digitally, safeguarding this information becomes a critical component of ethical therapy practice. Therapists must be vigilant about the digital tools they choose, ensuring they provide both robust security measures and ease of use for clients.

The use of digital tools also paves the way for enhanced continuity of care. For clients who relocate or have unpredictable schedules, technology ensures they can maintain therapy without disruption. Whether through video conferencing, digital check-ins, or accessing resources online, the flexibility offered by digital tools helps maintain therapeutic momentum and prevents loss of progress.

Furthermore, digital platforms can facilitate group therapy sessions, connecting clients from various geographical locations who share similar experiences. This connectivity fosters a sense of community and support among participants, crucial for those who may feel isolated in their healing journey. Group sessions conducted digitally can also alleviate some logistical concerns, such as travel and room availability, making group therapy more accessible and practical for therapists and clients alike.

The adoption of technology in CPT isn't merely about keeping up with the times; it's about enhancing the therapeutic process to make it more client- friendly and effective. Digital tools must be used thoughtfully and skillfully, ensuring they complement rather than replace the human aspects of therapy. They should be an extension of the therapist's expertise and empathy, not a substitute for these fundamental elements of care.

In conclusion, the integration of digital tools into CPT marks a transformative shift towards more flexible, data-driven, and client- centered therapeutic practices. As these technologies continue to evolve, they promise to offer richer resources, more precise treatment modalities, and broader access to effective care for all individuals seeking to overcome PTSD. Embracing these tools requires an open mind and a commitment to continuous learning, yet the rewards they offer in terms of improved client outcomes and enhanced therapeutic relationships are well worth the effort. The landscape of mental health care is expanding, and with it, the potential for truly transformative healing journeys powered by technology.

Teletherapy Considerations

The digital age has ushered in a transformative shift in how mental health services are delivered. As we integrate technology within Cognitive Processing Therapy (CPT), teletherapy emerges as a pivotal consideration for clinicians aiming to broaden access to care. The ability to engage with patients in a virtual space not only alleviates geographic and logistical barriers but also fosters a new kind of accessibility that many patients find appealing and beneficial.

Teletherapy provides a flexible framework for CPT delivery, making mental health care more accessible for those who might face obstacles in accessing traditional in-person therapy. Technological advancements enable therapists to meet clients where they are, offering convenience for patients with constrained schedules or mobility issues and those in remote areas without easy access to specialized mental health services. However, teletherapy is not without its challenges, creating a need for careful consideration and modification of typical treatment protocols.

One primary consideration when using teletherapy is ensuring patient privacy and confidentiality. Upholding these ethical obligations requires clinicians to use secure, HIPAA-compliant platforms for communication. Encryption protocols and two-factor authentication add layers of security, protecting sensitive patient data from potential breaches. It's crucial to discuss with patients the importance of maintaining a private and quiet space during sessions, much like they would in an office setting.

Teletherapy alters the dynamics of the therapeutic relationship. Eye contact might not be as direct, or body language may be more difficult to interpret through a screen. Therapists need to adapt their communication styles, perhaps amplifying their verbal cues or becoming more explicit in acknowledging patients' expressions and feelings. Although this modality challenges traditional nonverbal communication, it also offers a unique opportunity to deepen mutual understanding and empathy through focused and deliberate dialogue.

Setting boundaries becomes even more significant when working in a virtual format. The ease of access that teletherapy offers might inadvertently blur the lines between the therapist-patient relationship.

Therapists should establish clear expectations about session duration, frequency, and communication methods outside of scheduled appointments. Patients should be made aware of the importance of logging into sessions on time and ensuring that technical requirements, like stable internet connections, are met.

Cultural and individual considerations must also be taken into account. Adapting teletherapy methods to suit the diverse backgrounds and technological proficiency of patients is essential. Some may be uncomfortable or unfamiliar with teletherapy tools, requiring a more gradual introduction to the technology. Therapists can facilitate this process by providing instructions, conducting a test run before the first session, or even sending tutorial resources. For others, language barriers or different cultural norms regarding technology use might necessitate further adjustments.

Assessing and managing crises remotely poses another challenge in teletherapy. Whereas in-person interactions allow for immediate and tangible responses to crises, teletherapy requires therapists to have explicit protocols in place. Clinicians need to establish emergency contact procedures and ensure that patients know how to access local emergency services if need be. A shared safety plan developed at the onset of therapy can guide both the therapist and the patient through a range of emergency scenarios.

Teletherapy also invites innovative use of digital tools and resources to enhance CPT. Online platforms might offer interactive modules, homework assignments, and digital thought diaries that support the therapy process. These tools can encourage patients to actively engage with therapy materials between sessions, potentially leading to increased retention of therapeutic insights and greater overall progress.

The flexibility in scheduling and location can increase engagement and adherence to therapy. Patients who might otherwise miss sessions due to travel issues, illness, or childcare conflicts are more likely to keep their appointments. This continuity can contribute to better treatment outcomes. Therapists find that the convenience of conducting sessions from a home or office setting reduces cancellations and no-show rates compared to in- person therapy.

Feedback and progress evaluation in teletherapy remains crucial. Regular check-ins with patients about their comfort and satisfaction with the teletherapy format can uncover barriers that might impede therapeutic progress. Encouraging direct and open communication about what works and what doesn't helps tailor the therapy to meet each patient's unique needs. Progress should be evaluated with the same rigor as in face-to-face settings, ensuring that patient outcomes remain the focus.

In integrating teletherapy into CPT, it's important to remain aware of the ongoing advancements in technology and therapy methods. Continuous education on new telehealth regulations, technological tools, and emerging best practices is vital for therapists to stay effective and ethical in a rapidly evolving field. As the landscape of mental health care continues to shift, so too must the methods by which we offer healing and support.

Ultimately, the adoption of teletherapy into CPT offers both opportunities and challenges. With thoughtful application and adaptation, these digital methods can expand the reach of life-changing therapeutic interventions, making them accessible to a broader audience than ever before. The success of teletherapy hinges on our ability to blend the old with the new —merging traditional therapeutic principles with modern technological capabilities. In doing so, therapists not only uphold the standards of care but also catalyze a future where mental health support is within reach for all who seek it.

Ethical Implications

The integration of technology in Cognitive Processing Therapy (CPT) promises a wealth of enhancements in treatment accessibility and effectiveness, yet it also invites a host of ethical considerations that must be carefully examined. Delving into these ethical implications is crucial, as we're tasked with balancing innovation with the sanctity of patient well- being and therapeutic integrity.

One of the primary ethical concerns when integrating technology into CPT revolves around confidentiality and privacy. The use of digital tools such as mobile apps, online platforms, and teletherapy inherently involves data storage and transmission. Such technologies might heighten the risk of unauthorized access to sensitive information. Therapists and mental health professionals must ensure stringent data protection measures are in place, abiding by HIPAA guidelines and using encrypted communication methods to safeguard patient privacy. It's essential to communicate these digital boundaries clearly to patients, helping them understand how their data will be handled and protected.

Moreover, teletherapy raises questions about informed consent. With traditional face-to-face therapy sessions, there's a mutual understanding and nuance in non-verbal communication that might be lost or misinterpreted in digital formats. Therapists must ensure that patients fully comprehend what teletherapy entails, including potential risks such as miscommunication or technical issues. Consent should be an ongoing, dynamic process rather than a one-time formality, requiring continual dialogue and reassurance.

However, the technology's reach can be a double-edged sword. While it enables therapy access to geographically isolated or mobility-challenged individuals, it also opens up the potential for delivering therapy in regions with differing laws, cultural norms, and ethical standards. Therapists must navigate this delicate terrain by being culturally competent and aware of the legal frameworks governing psychological services in different areas. Adapting therapeutic techniques to fit cultural contexts without compromising quality care stands as a significant ethical responsibility.

Then comes the challenge of maintaining therapeutic presence and rapport through digital means. The screen's mediation can sometimes create feelings of depersonalization or detachment, impacting the therapeutic alliance's strength. A robust therapeutic relationship is critical in CPT, as it forms the foundation of trust and openness required for trauma processing. Professionals must be adept at using verbal cues and empathy to bridge this digital divide, ensuring patients feel truly seen and heard despite the virtual barrier.

Furthermore, technology in CPT can inadvertently affect the therapeutic process itself. Automation and digital interventions, while efficient, may risk oversimplifying complex human experiences into algorithmic interactions. This potential depersonalization could dilute the effectiveness of therapy, as it may not fully cater to the nuanced and individualized experiences of trauma survivors. It's crucial to remember that technology should augment—not replace—the deeply personal and relational aspects of therapy.

Additionally, there's the ethical dilemma of digital competence. Therapists must be not only technically proficient with the tools they employ but also capable of troubleshooting and managing any technological mishaps that might arise. Lack of such competence can disrupt the therapeutic process, potentially harming patient trust and engagement. Investing in training and staying updated with technological advancements becomes an ethical obligation for therapists wishing to offer tech-integrated CPT.

As we traverse this digital landscape, it's also imperative to consider equity in access. Not all patients may have the necessary resources or digital literacy to engage with tech-enabled services effectively. This digital divide could inadvertently marginalize certain populations, creating disparities in treatment access and outcomes. Mental health professionals should strive to offer alternatives that accommodate various levels of technological access and proficiency, ensuring no patient is left behind.

Finally, there's the question of over-reliance on technology. As the allure of technological convenience grows, there's a risk of veering towards mechanistic protocols at the expense of human intuition and empathy, which are indispensable in trauma therapy. Therapists should remain vigilant, constantly reflecting on their practice to ensure that technology serves as a tool, not a crutch, in delivering compassionate, person- centered care.

In conclusion, while integrating technology in CPT presents a plethora of opportunities to enhance therapeutic reach and efficacy, it compels us to tread carefully through an intricate web of ethical considerations. By reflecting on these implications and committing to ethical practices, we can harness technology's potential to empower patients while preserving the integrity and humanity of therapy.

CHAPTER 20

LONG-TERM MANAGEMENT STRATEGIES

As we transition into the realm of long-term management strategies, it's essential to underscore the resilience and dedication required to sustain progress in overcoming PTSD. For healthcare providers, the journey doesn't end with therapy sessions; it extends into crafting a sustainable framework that empowers patients to navigate life's challenges post- therapy. Relapse prevention emerges as a pivotal focus, necessitating the integration of personalized strategies tailored to each individual's unique experiences and recovery trajectory.

Sustaining progress involves reinforcing the cognitive and emotional tools patients have acquired, ensuring they remain vigilant in identifying early signs of distress, and bridging them with proper support resources. Whether it's fostering connections with support groups or utilizing technology-driven interventions, the goal is to cultivate a resilient network that reinforces treatment gains. It's imperative to adopt a mindset of proactive adaptation, where strategies evolve in tandem with an individual's growth, allowing for a seamless transition from therapist-guided sessions to patient-led empowerment. This chapter serves not merely as guidance but as a reminder that long-term management is a shared commitment between patient and practitioner, a thoughtful dance of empathy, innovation, and unwavering perseverance.

To truly sustain progress, it is essential to integrate ongoing learning and adaptation into the therapeutic process. Research has shown that individuals who actively engage in self-monitoring, such as using apps to track mood, stress levels, or triggers, are better able to recognize early signs of distress before they escalate. This proactive approach empowers patients to intervene early, utilizing coping strategies they have cultivated in therapy to manage potential setbacks. Furthermore, as patients continue their healing journey, their needs and coping strategies will inevitably evolve. Digital platforms, such as telehealth services or mobile therapy apps, allow for real-time adjustments to treatment plans, providing a bridge between in-person sessions and self-guided care. This flexibility not only supports continued growth but also helps patients feel more confident in managing their mental health long-term. By blending traditional therapeutic techniques with modern technological tools, mental health professionals can foster a robust, adaptable support system that empowers patients to confidently navigate their recovery with autonomy and resilience.

Relapse Prevention

Relapse prevention is a critical component of long-term management strategies in the treatment of PTSD. The journey of healing doesn't stop once initial therapy goals are met; it's an ongoing process that requires both vigilance and adaptability. The key is not just in alleviating symptoms temporarily but in equipping individuals with the tools to maintain their progress over the long haul. Relapse, while disheartening, can offer valuable insights that contribute to deeper understanding and resilience.

In practical terms, relapse prevention involves anticipating and managing potential setbacks. The foundation of this approach is rooted in empowerment, teaching individuals to recognize their own warning signs and to implement strategies proactively. This forward-thinking mindset fosters a sense of agency that can be particularly empowering for people who've often felt helpless in the grip of trauma.

One of the main strategies in relapse prevention is continuous self- monitoring. Encouraging individuals to keep regular check-ins with themselves can be incredibly beneficial. This might involve maintaining a journal or using self-assessment tools that track emotions, thoughts, and reactions. Such exercises not only promote self-awareness but also help detect early signs of relapse, enabling timely intervention.

Cognitive restructuring plays an equally crucial role in relapse prevention. By challenging maladaptive thoughts and reinforcing positive beliefs, individuals can cultivate a mental environment less conducive to relapse. Practicing mindfulness regularly can help reinforce these cognitive strategies by promoting present-focused awareness and reducing rumination.

Incorporating lifestyle changes is another pivotal aspect of relapse prevention. Encouraging patients to adopt healthy lifestyle habits can significantly lower the risk of relapse. Regular physical exercise, nutritious dieting, adequate sleep, and effective stress management techniques like meditation or yoga can positively impact mental health, making individuals more resilient against potential triggers.

The support network around the individual is another critical component. Creating and maintaining a strong network of friends, family, and colleagues who understand the journey and are supportive can serve as a buffer against relapse. These relationships can provide the reassurance and accountability necessary to stay on track when personal resolve might falter.

Healthcare providers need to be aware of their patients' specific challenges and triggers. By working collaboratively with patients, they can develop personalized relapse prevention plans that address unique stressors and environmental factors. This tailored approach is essential in acknowledging the diverse experiences of trauma survivors and respecting their individual pathways to recovery.

Relapse prevention involves setting realistic expectations for the recovery process. Patients need to understand that healing isn't a linear path, and setbacks aren't failures, but rather part of the journey. Healthcare providers play a crucial role in conveying this message, helping individuals shift their focus from an idealized, flawless recovery to one that embraces resilience and the capacity to rebound from setbacks.

Furthermore, ongoing education about PTSD and its management is a cornerstone of relapse prevention. Ensuring that patients are well- informed about their condition fosters a deeper understanding, making them better equipped to manage potential relapses.

Educational sessions can include topics such as recognizing warning signs, implementing coping strategies, and understanding the neurobiological aspects of PTSD, which can demystify the experience and reduce anxiety surrounding symptoms.

Crisis intervention plans can serve as a robust safety net in relapse prevention. These plans are pre-established procedures designed to be implemented when an individual feels they're approaching a critical point. They include steps like contacting a therapist or a trusted friend, visiting a healthcare facility if necessary, or engaging in pre-planned therapeutic activities.

Support groups or peer-led initiatives can act as valuable adjuncts to professional treatment plans. These groups offer a safe space for individuals to share experiences and strategies, gain new perspectives, and draw strength from shared experiences. The sense of belonging and mutual understanding inherent in these groups can have a therapeutic effect and play a critical role in relapse prevention efforts.

In terms of therapeutic interventions, cognitive-behavioral approaches have proven effective in reducing relapse rates. These techniques focus on modifying dysfunctional thinking patterns and behaviors, equipping individuals with coping strategies that empower them to manage stressors effectively.

Therapists must also maintain a degree of flexibility in their approach. As individuals progress in their recovery, their needs and circumstances may change, necessitating adaptations in the therapeutic plan. Regular follow- ups and reviews can help ensure that the treatment remains relevant and effective in preventing relapses.

Ultimately, successful relapse prevention is about fostering resilience. This involves not only mitigating risk factors but also enhancing protective factors. Practitioners should focus on building on patients' strengths, encouraging the development of new skills, and facilitating opportunities for positive growth. With a comprehensive and individualized relapse prevention plan, individuals can navigate their recovery journey with increased confidence and hope.

Sustaining Progress

Preserving progress gained through Cognitive Processing Therapy (CPT) isn't just an endpoint—it's a continuous journey. Once the core work of therapy is concluded, patients often find themselves on uncharted terrain. The skills and insights obtained during sessions must now be integrated into daily life, fostering resilience and promoting long-term well-being. The essence of sustaining progress lies in the practice of new skills and the reinforcement of healthier cognitive patterns.

The transition from structured therapy sessions to the autonomy of everyday life can be daunting for many patients. Without the regular rhythm of appointments and the immediate availability of a supportive professional, individuals might find themselves yearning for guidance or reassurance. This is where the strategies learned in therapy come into play. By applying cognitive restructuring techniques independently, patients can counter lapses into maladaptive thought patterns, maintaining the cognitive gains achieved during therapy.

One important aspect of sustaining progress is the ongoing challenging of beliefs. It's critical for individuals to continue scrutinizing how they interpret the world and manage their experiences. Through self- assessment, they can identify distortions and consciously choose more adaptive beliefs. Encouraging patients to engage in reflective practices, such as journaling, can help them track their mental state and recognize shifts that indicate either growth or areas needing attention.

Social support plays a pivotal role in sustaining progress. Having a community or network to lean on can provide the social validation necessary for long-term recovery. Whether it's family, friends, or support groups, these connections offer ongoing encouragement and reinforcements of positive changes. They serve as reminders that patients are not alone in their journey, creating an environment where growth is nurtured and celebrated.

Moreover, relapse prevention can't be overlooked; it's a critical element in sustaining progress. By anticipating potential triggers and devising proactive strategies, patients equip themselves against setbacks. This preparedness includes recognizing early warning signs of cognitive or emotional downturns and having a plan ready to address them. Utilizing practical tools, such as emergency coping strategies and structured routines, can provide a safety net, bolstering confidence and reinforcing resilience.

Integrating technology could also bolster sustaining progress efforts by offering patients continuous access to therapeutic resources. Digital platforms, whether they embed apps, online support groups, or teletherapy sessions, can fill the void between formal therapy and the demands of independent living. They offer flexibility and convenience, ensuring patients have the support they need anytime and anywhere.

Ultimately, sustaining progress requires a sense of ownership over the therapeutic journey. Patients must see themselves as active agents in maintaining their mental health. Encouraging self-efficacy fosters a belief in their capacity to manage future challenges. This empowerment allows individuals to build upon their progress, continuously evolving beyond the confines of therapy.

In the grand scheme of recovery, sustaining progress stands as a testament to the enduring power of transformation. It's about cultivating a life that honors the lessons learned in therapy while remaining open to growth and change. With the foundation laid and strategies in place, individuals can navigate the complexities of life with greater resilience and an unwavering sense of hope.

Support Resources

In the journey of long-term management for individuals coping with PTSD, having the right support resources in place can make a significant difference. Support isn't just a luxury; it's a cornerstone for sustaining progress and preventing relapse. Just as a bridge needs both sturdy pillars and cables to hold up, so does someone navigating the complexities of trauma recovery. Let's delve into the types of support resources that can be crucial in this process.

First and foremost, community support should be acknowledged as a powerful resource. For many, connecting with others who've shared similar experiences can be profoundly healing. Peer support groups offer a unique space where individuals can exchange stories, challenges, and triumphs. These groups not only provide a sense of belonging and understanding but also reduce feelings of isolation by creating a network of shared experiences. Utilizing community centers, forums, or even online platforms dedicated to PTSD support can be immensely beneficial for those seeking collective strength.

In addition to community-based resources, professional support remains critical. Therapists specializing in trauma and PTSD are key allies in maintaining therapeutic gains. Regular check-ins, either in one-on-one sessions or group therapy, can help keep individuals on track with their recovery goals. Participating in "booster" sessions even after the initial therapy period concludes can fortify insights and skills acquired during treatment, helping individuals navigate the ebb and flow of everyday life.

Furthermore, the guidance of mental health professionals isn't limited to traditional in-person sessions. The increasing integration of technology into therapeutic practices has expanded access to resources significantly. Digital tools like teletherapy and mental health apps can offer continuous support and monitoring, providing individuals with remote access to their therapists and self-help resources at their fingertips. This approach not only offers flexibility but also addresses barriers like geographical limitations and scheduling conflicts.

Family support also plays a pivotal role in long-term management. Educating family members about PTSD can foster empathy and understanding, transforming them into adept supporters. It's essential for families to be involved in the treatment process when appropriate, as they can help reinforce coping strategies and provide emotional backing during challenging times. Family therapy sessions can be instrumental in rebuilding relationships that might have been strained by trauma-related issues.

In some cases, spiritual or faith-based resources might offer significant support. For many, spirituality can provide a framework for meaning- making and resilience, which is enriching to the recovery process.

Engaging with spiritual advisors or participating in faith communities can provide comfort and a sense of purpose, helping individuals to feel grounded and hopeful about the future.

Moreover, educational resources should not be overlooked as a form of support. Knowledge encourages empowerment, enabling individuals to take control of their recovery journey. Access to quality educational materials that explain the intricacies of PTSD and its management can motivate individuals to actively engage in self-help practices. Providing resources like books, workshops, and online courses can help individuals and their support networks deepen their understanding and refine their strategies for coping with PTSD.

Healthcare providers should also consider the value of creating a comprehensive resource directory. Such a directory can be a vital tool for both patients and practitioners, listing available local and online support groups, mental health professionals, telehealth services, emergency contacts, and educational materials. Having this information readily available can streamline the process for practitioners advocating for a multi-faceted support approach, while giving patients the autonomy to explore options that best meet their needs.

Additionally, building a multidisciplinary support network can enhance the effectiveness of long-term management strategies. Collaboration between psychiatrists, psychologists, social workers, occupational therapists, and other professionals can offer a holistic view of recovery that addresses various aspects of a patient's life. Regular interdisciplinary meetings can ensure all care providers are aligned, providing consistent support that tackles both mental health needs and social or physical challenges.

Ultimately, equipping individuals with a diverse arsenal of support resources creates a robust safety net that can absorb setbacks and promote resilience. The key to effective long-term management of PTSD involves acknowledging the necessity of support and integrating diverse resources that address emotional, social, and physical needs. By prioritizing support systems that align with individual preferences and lifestyles, health care providers can empower individuals to not just manage their symptoms but to thrive in life beyond trauma.

CHAPTER 21

TAILORING CPT FOR VETERANS

In working with veterans, tailoring Cognitive Processing Therapy (CPT) requires a deep understanding of military culture and the unique traumas often experienced by those who have served. Veterans might carry memories from combat, deployments, or other military-related experiences that can profoundly shape their beliefs and reactions.

Effective interventions in CPT for veterans involve acknowledging the discipline and camaraderie that mark military life while helping them process traumatic memories and challenge maladaptive thoughts that arise. Providers must foster a therapeutic space that respects the resilience inherent in military experiences and adapts therapeutic techniques to honor that strength. This tailored approach not only addresses the specific narrative and emotional needs of veterans but also empowers them to reintegrate into civilian life with renewed hope and agency.

An essential component of tailoring CPT for veterans is recognizing the often complex and layered nature of military trauma, which can include moral injury, survivor's guilt, and the psychological effects of combat-related stress. Studies show that veterans frequently struggle with the transition from military to civilian life, as they must reconcile their service experiences with the expectations and realities of post-service life. This internal conflict can complicate the therapeutic process, making it crucial for providers to create an environment of understanding and trust. By integrating military culture into the therapeutic dialogue—acknowledging the veteran's sense of duty, sacrifice, and the bonds formed with fellow service members—therapists can build a rapport that honors the veteran's identity. Tailoring CPT to address these unique aspects of military service not only helps veterans process trauma but also empowers them to find strength in their experiences, viewing their past struggles as part of their broader narrative of resilience and survival. As research indicates, veterans who feel understood in the context of their service are more likely to engage in therapy and make meaningful progress toward healing and reintegration.

Understanding Military Culture

In order to effectively tailor Cognitive Processing Therapy (CPT) for veterans, it's crucial to first understand the unique culture of the military. The military ecosystem is built on traditions, hierarchies, and values that instill a sense of duty and camaraderie among its members. This environment, while supportive and structured, also presents unique psychological challenges that must be comprehended by health care providers and mental health professionals when addressing PTSD and other trauma-related conditions.

Military culture is deeply embedded in a framework of discipline and order. It's an institution where the chain of command holds significant sway, impacting not just decisions but also daily interactions. Unlike the civilian world, where personal freedom is more prioritized, military life requires conformity to rules and directives. This rigid structure, while essential for operational success, can sometimes lead to stressors that aren't immediately visible to those outside of this community.

Additionally, the sense of belonging among military personnel often transcends that of ordinary team-based environments. The shared experiences—be it training, peacekeeping missions, or combat operations—forge tight-knit bonds. Veterans often describe a profound loyalty to their units, viewing them as family. This sense of brotherhood or sisterhood can act as both a protective factor and a barrier. When engaging in therapy, therapists need to recognize these bonds and consider how they affect a veteran's willingness to engage in therapeutic processes that may seem alien or unnecessary from their perspective.

The impact of military culture extends to communication styles as well. Veterans might display a different approach when discussing personal experiences, often using jargon or acronyms that are second nature within their circles but may be opaque to outsiders. The act of expressing vulnerability can feel contrary to what they've been conditioned to show— a challenge when discussing traumatic memories. As therapists, developing a keen awareness of these communication nuances is essential. Engaging with veterans involves not only understanding their terminology but appreciating the context in which such terms operate.

Another critical aspect to consider is the notion of stoicism. Service members are often revered for their ability to maintain composure under pressure. This cultural expectation can lead some veterans to minimize or underreport psychological distress or trauma symptoms, fearing they might be perceived as weak or incapable. Mental health professionals working with this population must navigate these deeply rooted beliefs with sensitivity, encouraging open dialogue while respecting the veteran's pace and comfort level.

The transition from military to civilian life presents its own unique challenges. Veterans may struggle with the loss of identity tied to their service roles. In the military, roles and responsibilities are clearly defined, and each individual's contribution is part of a larger mission. The abrupt shift to civilian life can result in a loss of purpose or direction, leading to feelings of isolation or disorientation. This aspect plays a substantial role in therapy, where assisting veterans in redefining their sense of purpose is crucial to their healing and reintegration process.

When tailoring CPT for veterans, acknowledging the influence of military culture on family dynamics is equally vital. Military families often experience significant sacrifices—from frequent relocations to extended deployments—all of which contribute to unique stressors. These experiences can affect family relationships and dynamics, which may need to be explored in therapy. Including family members in the therapeutic process when appropriate can enhance understanding and support for veterans.

Beyond individual and familial considerations, therapists should also be familiar with the broader societal perceptions of military service.

Veterans often contend with misunderstanding or stereotypical perceptions from civilians, which may contribute to a sense of alienation. Recognizing this external pressure can aid therapists in developing strategies that foster community integration and resilience-building for veterans.

Ultimately, understanding military culture is not about viewing it as a monolith but appreciating its nuances and the way these influence the lived experiences of veterans. Each individual's journey is distinct, shaped by personal memories and interpretations of their service time. By delving deeper into the cultural aspects that define military life, mental health professionals can forge empathic and effective therapeutic relationships, offering services that truly resonate with this unique population. Through compassion, curiosity, and cultural competency, therapists can guide veterans in reclaiming their mental space and navigating the complexities that arise from their service. This not only aids in individual recovery but contributes to a broader understanding and appreciation of the sacrifices made by those who have served.

Common Traumas in Veterans

When tailoring Cognitive Processing Therapy (CPT) for veterans, understanding the specific traumas they frequently encounter is crucial. Military service, by its very nature, exposes individuals to experiences that are both challenging and potentially traumatic. While no two service members' experiences are identical, there are patterns in the types of trauma that veterans most commonly report. These experiences can significantly influence both the presentation of PTSD and the therapeutic approaches that may be most effective.

Combat exposure is perhaps the most well-known source of trauma among veterans. The realities of battle—a constant threat to life, witnessing death, and the need to make split-second decisions under duress—can leave lasting psychological scars. Many veterans contend with memories of intense firefights, the loss of comrades, or injuries sustained in the line of duty. These experiences can contribute to symptoms such as hyper-vigilance, intrusive thoughts, and emotional numbing. For healthcare providers, it's critical to appreciate how these experiences shape veterans' worldviews, often altering their core beliefs about safety, trust, and control.

However, combat is not the only source of trauma for veterans. Military Sexual Trauma (MST) is another significant issue affecting both male and female service members. MST encompasses any sexual harassment or assault that occurs in military settings. The deeply hierarchical nature of military culture can compound the trauma, creating environments where victims might feel unable to report their experiences without fear of retaliation or disbelief. As a result, addressing MST in therapy requires an emphasis on safety, validation, and empowerment, recognizing the unique barriers these survivors face in seeking help.

Additionally, deployment-related stressors extend beyond the battlefield. Veterans often endure significant separations from family, post- deployment reintegration challenges, and the pressures of adjusting to "normal" life after military service. These stressors can exacerbate existing psychological conditions or contribute to the development of new ones. The dissonance between military and civilian life can be jarring, with veterans sometimes struggling to find a sense of purpose or belonging upon returning home. Therapists must remain acutely aware of these challenges when designing treatment plans, ensuring that they address both the immediate symptoms of trauma and the broader context of the veteran's life.

It's also essential to consider the impact of moral injury, a lesser-known but equally critical concept in veteran trauma. Moral injury occurs when individuals violate their own ethical or moral codes, often under the extreme conditions of war. Veterans might grapple with guilt or shame related to actions taken in combat or the perceived failure to prevent harm. Unlike PTSD, moral injury is less about fear and more about a profound sense of remorse or disillusionment. Effective therapy, therefore, involves facilitating processes of forgiveness, meaning- making, and acceptance. Understanding the nuances of moral injury can enhance the therapist's ability to create a compassionate and non- judgmental therapeutic space.

Another dimension of veteran trauma involves the role of leadership and authority within the military structure. Experiences of betrayal by trusted leaders or the system can deeply affect a service member's psyche. Whether due to perceived neglect or outright abuse of power, these situations can leave veterans with feelings of abandonment and mistrust toward institutions. Addressing these experiences in therapy involves rebuilding trust, both within the therapeutic relationship and, more broadly, in the veteran's life outside of treatment.

The compounded nature of these traumas often requires a multifaceted approach to therapy, one that accommodates the complexities of military service. CPT can provide a structured yet flexible framework that allows for the exploration of cognitive distortions, the rewriting of trauma narratives, and the cultivation of resilience. By understanding the specific traumas that veterans endure, clinicians can offer interventions that not only alleviate symptoms but also facilitate a deeper integration of the veteran's traumatic experiences into their personal narratives, promoting healing and growth.

In summary, a decisive step in tailoring CPT for veterans is the nuanced understanding of common traumas—combat, MST, moral injury, and system betrayal among them. These experiences, while universally challenging, can also be deeply personal and unique. By crafting a therapy that honors both the shared and individual elements of veteran trauma, mental health professionals can help dismantle the barriers that keep veterans from reclaiming their time and mental space. This, ultimately, is the heart of therapeutic work: empowering veterans to reshape their narratives and embrace a future redefined by resilience and understanding.

Effective Interventions

When working with veterans in Cognitive Processing Therapy (CPT), the effectiveness of interventions largely depends on a nuanced understanding of military culture, individual experiences, and the specific traumas faced by this population. Addressing these factors not only enhances therapeutic outcomes but also builds trust and rapport, enabling meaningful healing journeys. Veterans often carry distinct experiences that shape their worldviews and belief systems. Tailoring interventions in CPT involves acknowledging this uniqueness while addressing the common themes of guilt, betrayal, and loss that many veterans face.

A critical component of effective interventions is recognizing the distinct cognitive schemas that veterans develop during military service. These schemas, influenced by principles such as duty, honor, and sacrifice, may clash with civilian life, leading to cognitive dissonance and emotional distress. Thus, customizing CPT to align with or gently challenge these schemas can make therapy more relatable and impactful. For instance, exploring the dichotomy between military valor and the civilian perception of vulnerability can help veterans reconstruct their beliefs without feeling invalidated.

In CPT, addressing avoidance behavior is essential. Veterans often engage in avoidance to shield themselves from overwhelming emotions related to traumatic events. Effective interventions focus on gently encouraging veterans to confront these emotions within a safe environment. Facilitating gradual exposure through trauma narratives helps veterans process and integrate their traumatic experiences, reducing the impact of avoidance on their daily functioning. This process not only aids in desensitizing the trauma but also empowers veterans to regain control over intrusive memories and thoughts.

Alongside narrative exposure, cognitive restructuring is a vital intervention. Challenging maladaptive beliefs rooted in trauma is essential in modifying perceptions of self and world. For veterans, this may mean addressing beliefs such as "I failed my comrades" or "I am unworthy of love." By collaboratively reevaluating these beliefs, veterans can shift towards more adaptive, realistic cognitions, promoting a healthier self-concept and improved interpersonal relationships.

Addressing guilt and shame is another crucial aspect of effective interventions for veterans. These emotions, often stemming from moral injury or perceived failures, can be debilitating. Interventions that facilitate compassion-focused therapy within the CPT framework can be immensely beneficial. Encouraging veterans to engage in self- forgiveness practices, and aiding them in distinguishing between guilt and responsibility, allows for emotional healing and reduced self- condemnation. This process involves nurturing empathy and self- compassion, which are crucial in overcoming the pervasive guilt that many veterans experience.

Moreover, peer support can significantly enhance the effectiveness of CPT interventions for veterans. Group CPT sessions, where veterans can share their experiences and insights, foster a sense of community and understanding. This shared space offers validation and decreases the isolation many veterans feel in civilian environments. Drawing from the collective strength of military camaraderie, these sessions encourage veterans to support each other while working through their challenges.

Integrating holistic approaches, such as mindfulness and relaxation techniques, can also complement traditional CPT interventions. Veterans may benefit from learning skills that promote present-moment awareness, reducing the reactivity to distressing memories or thoughts. Techniques like deep breathing, progressive muscle relaxation, and guided imagery serve as adjunctive interventions that help veterans manage stress and anxiety, thereby enhancing their emotional resilience throughout the therapy process.

Incorporating family involvement can further optimize CPT interventions. Veterans' families play a significant role in their recovery journey. Educating families about PTSD and promoting open communication can reduce misunderstandings and foster supportive environments. In certain cases, involving family members in therapy sessions can enhance understanding and cohesion, allowing veterans to feel supported in their recovery.

Furthermore, considering physical health is crucial in this context. Many veterans face physical injuries alongside psychological trauma.

Collaborating with healthcare professionals to address both domains— and ensuring continuity of care across physical and mental health services —can help create a comprehensive treatment approach. Recognizing the interplay between physical and mental well-being is vital in effective intervention strategies.

Adaptation of CPT materials and language is another important consideration. Therapy materials should reflect military terms and scenarios relevant to veterans' experiences. This approach facilitates greater engagement and ensures that interventions resonate with the challenges faced during and after service. Clinicians should be familiar with military terminology and cultural nuances to communicate effectively, thereby maximizing therapeutic rapport and progress.

Ultimately, effective interventions in CPT for veterans demand a compassionate, culturally sensitive, and multifaceted approach. By honoring veterans' experiences and adapting therapeutic strategies to meet their unique needs, mental health professionals can significantly impact the healing journey. Through tailored interventions, veterans can navigate their paths to recovery, reclaiming their lives and redefining their narratives with strength and resilience.

CHAPTER
22

ADAPTING CPT FOR CHILDREN AND ADOLESCENTS

Adapting Cognitive Processing Therapy for children and adolescents requires a deep understanding of their unique developmental stages and the ability to engage them effectively within their social environments. Unlike adults, younger individuals process trauma and therapy differently, demanding techniques that are both age-appropriate and sensitive to their cognitive and emotional growth.

To facilitate healing, it's crucial to incorporate playful and interactive elements that inspire engagement and resilience. Empowering families with tools and strategies is also essential, as it ensures a supportive home environment that reinforces therapeutic progress. By fostering a collaborative atmosphere that includes family members, therapists can harness the strength of familial bonds, enabling children and adolescents to feel supported throughout their journey.

Importantly, adapting CPT for this demographic calls for creativity and flexibility, encouraging mental health professionals to innovate within the bounds of evidence-based practice. In doing so, we not only tailor therapy to their needs but also instill hope and empowerment, nurturing the seeds of resilience and recovery.

Incorporating playful and interactive elements into therapy for children and adolescents can significantly enhance their engagement and emotional processing. Research shows that when therapy includes creative activities—such as art, storytelling, or role-playing—young patients are often more open to discussing difficult emotions and experiences. These activities allow children to express themselves in ways that might be more comfortable and accessible than traditional talk therapy. Moreover, such methods help reinforce the cognitive and emotional tools they are learning, making them feel more empowered and confident in managing their emotions. Playful techniques also encourage a sense of agency, allowing children to feel active in their healing process rather than passive recipients of treatment. This approach aligns well with CPT, as it enables children to challenge maladaptive thoughts and process trauma in a safe, structured, and engaging environment.

Equally important is the involvement of family members, as they play a vital role in maintaining therapeutic progress and supporting resilience. By educating families on trauma-informed care and providing them with practical tools—such as communication strategies and coping mechanisms—therapists can help create a consistent and supportive environment at home. Studies have shown that when families are actively involved in the therapeutic process, children and adolescents tend to experience faster recovery and greater emotional stability.

This collaborative approach not only enhances the child's treatment experience but also helps family members develop a deeper understanding of trauma and its impact. When families unite in support, they become a source of strength, reinforcing the therapeutic progress made in sessions and helping children feel safe and validated throughout their healing journey.

Developmental Considerations

Children and adolescents are not merely miniature adults; their cognitive, emotional, and social development requires a nuanced approach when adapting Cognitive Processing Therapy (CPT). Understanding the developmental stage of a child is crucial because it informs how they process trauma, articulate their experiences, and engage in therapeutic interventions. Typically, children possess a more concrete style of thinking, whereas adolescents begin to display more abstract reasoning. This transformation affects how they interpret events, sense of self, and their capacity for empathy and perspective-taking.

Therapists need to consider the developmental milestones relevant to the age group they're working with. For younger children, therapy may need to revolve more around play and creative expression rather than traditional talking therapies. Play therapy can become a vital tool here, offering a window into the child's thoughts and feelings in a way that more structured exercises cannot. It allows children to express what they might not yet have the language for, providing them with a narrative form that's both natural and accessible.

Adolescents, on the other hand, often seek autonomy and privacy, which can lead to reluctance in sharing their trauma experiences. The therapist's role shifts slightly to address these growth issues. There's an opportunity to encourage adolescents to take ownership of their therapy process, which can be empowering and convey respect for their emerging adult identity. Engaging them in the process of setting therapeutic goals is one way to validate their sense of agency.

It's also important to consider the cognitive load that CPT activities can place on a young person. With school, extracurricular activities, and sometimes part-time jobs, adolescents' schedules can be demanding. Therefore, the pacing and timing of therapy sessions must be flexible enough to fit within their existing commitments, minimizing additional stress. Effective therapists will be adept at balancing structured interventions with the spontaneous needs that arise during adolescence—a period characterized by rapid and sometimes tumultuous changes.

Emotion regulation is another area where developmental considerations are significant. Younger age groups may not have the vocabulary or emotional understanding to label what they're feeling. Therefore, therapists can implement tools such as emotion cards or visual aids to help children articulate and process their emotions. It can be a simple yet profound way to build emotional literacy, laying a foundation that will serve them throughout their lives.

Social dynamics play a crucial role as well. Peer relationships are paramount, particularly for adolescents. The therapist must navigate the impact of these relationships on a young person's self-esteem and well- being. Group CPT sessions can be an effective way to harness the power of peer acceptance and communal understanding for healing, albeit requiring careful management to protect confidentiality and maintain a safe environment.

Family dynamics are an additional layer of consideration. Families often play an integral role in the therapeutic process for children and adolescents. Involving a supportive family can provide a solid framework for reinforcing skills learned in therapy. Nevertheless, the therapist has to be sensitive to complex family systems, respecting boundaries while promoting an environment where open communication and healing can take place.

One must also pay attention to cultural and environmental factors that may influence how children and adolescents experience trauma and therapy. Cultural sensitivity isn't just about understanding a child's background—it involves incorporating these insights into the therapy process. Tailoring interventions to best meet the cultural needs of the child can support more effective and resonant outcomes.

Lastly, therapists should be cognizant of the importance of resilience and plasticity in younger individuals. Children and adolescents have an incredible capacity for change. Therapeutic interventions can not only help them recover from trauma but also assist them in developing vital life skills that contribute to their resilience. Cultivating an environment where young clients feel safe to explore experiences and emotions provides the foundational encouragement they need to rebuild their narrative in a more adaptive manner.

Cultural and environmental factors play a pivotal role in how children and adolescents perceive and process trauma. For instance, children from immigrant families or marginalized communities may experience additional layers of stress due to acculturation challenges, discrimination, or a lack of accessible mental health resources. Research shows that culturally adapted therapies—those that respect and integrate a child's cultural values, beliefs, and practices—can lead to more positive therapeutic outcomes. This approach might involve incorporating culturally relevant metaphors, traditions, or family dynamics into treatment, allowing the therapy process to resonate more deeply with the child. Moreover, therapists should be mindful of any potential barriers that may prevent families from seeking help, such as language differences, stigma surrounding mental health, or economic challenges. By addressing these factors with cultural competence and sensitivity, therapists can foster a more inclusive and effective therapeutic environment, making it easier for young clients to feel understood and supported in their healing journey.

In addition to cultural sensitivity, the inherent resilience and neuroplasticity of younger individuals offer a unique opportunity for growth through therapy. Neuroscience research consistently demonstrates that children and adolescents have an incredible ability to rewire their brains and develop new coping mechanisms, even after experiencing trauma. This plasticity means that, with the right interventions, children can not only recover from traumatic experiences but also emerge with enhanced emotional intelligence, problem-solving skills, and coping strategies. By fostering a therapeutic space that encourages curiosity and exploration, therapists can empower children to develop these life skills, promoting long-term resilience and emotional well-being. As children process trauma, they are not merely returning to a baseline state but are often growing in ways that enhance their ability to navigate life's challenges. The combination of cultural sensitivity, resilience, and therapeutic support provides a powerful foundation for young clients to rebuild their narratives and cultivate lasting strength.

Engaging Families

Engaging families in the therapeutic process is a crucial element when adapting Cognitive Processing Therapy (CPT) for children and adolescents. Involving family members not only provides critical support for the young individual but also creates an ecosystem within which healing and growth can thrive. The presence, understanding, and active participation of family members can reinforce the therapeutic journey and alleviate the pressures faced by the young patient navigating through trauma.

One of the first steps in engaging families involves psychoeducation. Helping families understand the impact of trauma and the principles behind CPT demystifies the process, enabling them to better support their child. Psychoeducation sessions should be tailored to illustrate that trauma can disrupt normal development and that therapy seeks to address these disruptions by targeting the underlying cognitive processes. The aim is to create an environment where families feel informed, involved, and empowered to assist their children.

Involving families isn't without its challenges. Diverse family dynamics, cultural backgrounds, and varying levels of stigma regarding mental health can influence engagement. It's essential to approach each family with sensitivity and understanding. Therapists should strive to build trust and offer a space where family members feel comfortable expressing their concerns and hopes. Emphasizing the family's role as an ally in therapy, rather than as a distant observer, can transform their engagement from passive to active participation.

Communication serves as a foundational tool for engaging families. Open, honest, and clear communication paves the way for effective collaboration. It's vital to establish a routine for family sessions and communication updates so that members are regularly informed about progress and challenges. This continuous dialogue helps to align therapeutic goals and family expectations, making the journey a collective effort rather than an isolated quest.

Empathy and validation are central to engaging families. Each family member may have their own emotional reactions and perceptions of the trauma and therapy. Providing a space for these emotions to be acknowledged and validated by the therapist can build rapport and understanding. This empathetic approach reinforces the therapeutic alliance, demonstrating that therapy is a collaborative effort that respects the experiences and emotions of everyone involved.

Family sessions can sometimes become emotionally charged, with underlying tensions surfacing. It is during these times that a therapist's skill in conflict resolution becomes invaluable. Guiding the family through these difficult discussions by facilitating healthy communication and encouraging mutual support can transform potential conflict into growth opportunities. Encouraging families to adopt a strengths-based perspective allows members to appreciate each individual's contributions to the healing process.

When families are engaged, they become co-architects of successful therapy outcomes. Encouraging them to share their insights about their child's progress and any changes they observe bridges the gap between clinical settings and home environments. Families can provide valuable feedback and suggest practical adaptations that can make therapy more relevant and impactful for the child's unique context.

It's also crucial to adapt engagement strategies as the child progresses through different developmental stages. A strategy that resonates with the family of an adolescent may differ from what's needed for a younger child. Therapists should remain flexible and responsive, adapting their approaches to reflect the evolving needs and capacities of the child and family. Such responsiveness not only fosters a supportive environment but showcases an understanding of the dynamic nature of child development.

Involving siblings and extended family members, when appropriate, can bolster the support framework. They often play significant roles in the child's life and can offer unique perspectives and support that complement the therapeutic processes. Including them in sessions or educational seminars can enhance their understanding and contribute to a more comprehensive family support network.

Finally, empowering families involves equipping them with the tools and strategies to foster resilience and support long-term healing. This includes teaching coping strategies, reinforcing positive communication patterns, and fostering an environment that prioritizes emotional and psychological well-being. The effects of trauma extend beyond the individual, and by engaging the family, therapists can help reshuffle familial patterns to create a nurturing space conducive to recovery.

Engaging families in CPT for children and adolescents is not only beneficial but essential. It represents a holistic approach that acknowledges the interconnectedness of family dynamics and individual healing. By prioritizing education, communication, empathy, and adaptability, therapists can transform family's involvement from being mere participants to becoming integral allies in the therapeutic journey, ensuring that healing is a collective endeavor.

Child-Specific Techniques

Children and adolescents require unique adaptations in Cognitive Processing Therapy (CPT) to meet their developmental needs and cognitive styles. Their understanding of trauma and its implications may differ significantly from adults, necessitating a sensitive and nuanced approach. For these younger individuals, trauma can pervade not just memories but also influence their developing belief systems and emotional regulation. Therefore, it's crucial to introduce CPT in a way that resonates with their experiences and cognitive capacities.

A tailored approach begins with adjusting the language and psychoeducation materials used in CPT. Younger clients benefit from simplified explanations of concepts like trauma and maladaptive thoughts. This can mean using metaphors and analogies relevant to their world. For instance, comparing trauma responses to a 'smoke detector' that goes off too easily can help children visualize and understand their heightened emotional states. The goal is to make complex psychological processes accessible without diluting their essence.

Engaging in therapeutic activities that tap into play and creativity is another effective child-specific technique. Play therapy, for example, is not only enjoyable but can be crucial in helping children express thoughts and emotions that they may not yet have the language for. Integrating activities such as drawing, storytelling, and role-playing enables the child to articulate their experiences in a non-threatening environment. These methods provide insight into their internal world, offering a bridge to more structured CPT interventions.

Developing a trauma narrative, a central component of CPT, requires careful adaptation for children. Instead of writing lengthy accounts, which might be intimidating or developmentally inappropriate, therapists can break this task into smaller, more manageable parts. Creating visual storyboards or utilizing narrative drawings allow children to convey their experiences at a comfortable pace. These exercises not only facilitate the expression of trauma but also empower children to reconstruct their experiences into coherent narratives.

Understanding the role of family in the therapy process is another fundamental aspect to consider. Families are part of the child's ecosystem and often play a significant role in the recovery journey. Engaging family members in psychoeducation can help them understand the therapy's purpose and the impact of trauma on the child. It's also important to guide families in supporting the child outside of therapy, ensuring consistency in addressing trauma-related symptoms and behaviors.

Emotional regulation is another area where children often need additional support and strategies tailored to their developmental stage. Simple mindfulness exercises and breathing techniques can be introduced to help them manage overwhelming emotions. For younger children, incorporating physical activities or games that focus on self-regulation can be particularly effective. By making these techniques fun and engaging, children are more likely to integrate them into their daily lives.

Incorporating caregiver involvement in sessions can further bolster therapeutic outcomes. This can include joint sessions or periodic updates where the therapist, child, and caregiver collaborate to refine coping strategies and therapy goals. This involvement not only supports the child but also strengthens the caregiver-child relationship, which can be affected by trauma.

Finally, therapists must remain flexible, adapting interventions based on the child's feedback and progress. Regular check-ins with the child about what is working or what feels challenging can guide therapy adjustments. This collaborative approach helps maintain engagement and enhances the child's sense of agency in their healing process.

Adapting CPT for children and adolescents requires a compassionate, flexible approach that respects their unique developmental needs. By tailoring interventions to their cognitive level, integrating play and family involvement, therapists can create a supportive therapeutic environment where healing can truly flourish. This approach doesn't just address trauma but also fosters resilience, equipping young individuals with skills for emotional processing and adaptive thinking that will benefit them long into adulthood.

Engaging caregivers in therapy sessions has been shown to significantly enhance the therapeutic process for children and adolescents, especially when trauma has strained family dynamics. When caregivers actively participate in therapy, they gain a deeper understanding of the child's emotional and psychological needs, learning how to provide consistent support and reinforce coping strategies at home. Research indicates that family involvement in therapy can lead to improved communication, emotional connection, and mutual understanding between caregivers and children, which in turn promotes better outcomes. For children, knowing that their caregivers are part of their healing process fosters a sense of security and stability, making them feel supported and validated in their journey. Joint sessions or updates allow therapists to address any concerns caregivers might have while providing a platform for the child to express their thoughts in the presence of trusted adults, creating an integrated support system that nurtures recovery on multiple fronts.

Additionally, the importance of flexibility in therapy cannot be overstated, particularly when working with younger individuals who are still developing emotional regulation and cognitive processing skills. Children and adolescents often experience rapid changes in their feelings, perceptions, and coping abilities, so regular check-ins with the child are crucial in adjusting interventions to better suit their evolving needs. This approach not only ensures that therapy remains relevant and effective but also allows the child to feel heard and empowered. Studies suggest that when children feel like active participants in their treatment, they are more likely to engage fully and commit to the process. Furthermore, by adapting interventions in response to the child's feedback, therapists can strengthen the therapeutic alliance, reinforcing trust and fostering a sense of collaboration. This dynamic, responsive approach ensures that the therapeutic environment remains supportive, flexible, and attuned to the unique needs of each child, ultimately fostering resilience and equipping them with valuable life skills for navigating future challenges.

CHAPTER 23

CONTINUING EDUCATION FOR THERAPISTS

Staying current and competent as a therapist involves more than just initial training; it requires a commitment to lifelong learning and professional growth. In the ever-evolving landscape of trauma therapy, continuing education is the cornerstone for maintaining effectiveness and delivering the highest standard of care. It's essential for therapists to engage in ongoing training opportunities, such as workshops, conferences, and online courses, to stay abreast of advancements in trauma-informed practices and emerging research.

These educational pursuits not only bolster a therapist's CPT expertise but also empower them to integrate innovative techniques and insights into their work. This dedication to self- improvement reinforces resilience and provides therapists with the tools needed to nurture hope and healing in their clients, ultimately fostering a more profound therapeutic impact. As you expand your knowledge and skill set, remember that embracing continuous learning is not just beneficial but crucial in the quest to support those on their path to recovery.

Training Opportunities

In the field of mental health, where the landscape is ever-changing, continuing education stands as a pillar of professional growth and competency. For therapists dedicated to aiding those grappling with trauma, embracing training opportunities is not just beneficial—it's essential. These opportunities are varied and can transform practice by integrating fresh insights and cutting-edge techniques.

Therapists often begin with foundational education, but with time, the need to build upon this foundation becomes paramount. Attending workshops and seminars can offer immersive experiences where therapists engage directly with nuanced aspects of trauma therapy. These environments encourage not only learning but also networking with other professionals who can provide diverse perspectives and experiences.

Webinars have become increasingly popular as a flexible learning option. They allow therapists to deepen their understanding from the comfort of their own offices or homes. During webinars, experts typically cover a multitude of topics—from updates on

CPT methodologies to innovative strategies for patient engagement. These digital seminars also offer the chance for interactive Q&A sessions, which can be invaluable for clarifying complex concepts.

Furthermore, certification programs are a significant aspect of continued learning for therapists specializing in trauma. These programs often delve into advanced techniques and provide a structured avenue for therapists to assess and enhance their skills. Obtaining certification not only boosts a therapist's credentials but also reassures patients of their commitment to professional excellence.

It's crucial to stay abreast of advancements in trauma therapy. Peer- reviewed journals offer a treasure trove of knowledge where therapists can learn about the latest research findings and theoretical developments. Subscribing to leading journals keeps professionals intellectually

engaged and informed about evidence-based practices that may better serve their clients.

Reading is complemented by attending national and international conferences. These gatherings are not just about listening to speakers; they are dynamic forums for exchanging ideas and challenging existing paradigms in therapeutic practice. Conferences can be transformative, offering fresh insights and reinvigorating a therapist's approach to treatment.

Continuing education should also include clinical practice updates. Engaging in peer consultation groups strengthens therapeutic strategies through shared discussions and case studies. These groups serve as a sounding board for new ideas and a place to obtain constructive feedback. They foster a culture of continuous improvement and collaboration among peers.

Moreover, mentorship programs offer unparalleled opportunities for both seasoned and novice therapists. By pairing with experienced mentors, therapists gain from the wealth of experience and wisdom that can't be gleaned from textbooks alone. These relationships are mutually beneficial, fostering an environment of growth, inspiration, and support.

On a more individualized level, pursuing self-study initiatives is valuable. Many credible online platforms offer self-paced courses focused on various aspects of CPT and trauma-informed care. This avenue allows therapists to delve deeply into subjects of particular interest or need, on their schedules and at their own pace.

Cultural competence is another critical dimension of training that cannot be overlooked. Ensuring that a therapist is equipped to handle the nuanced needs of diverse client populations requires regular and dedicated cultural sensitivity training. Such initiatives help therapists adapt their techniques and approaches to be more inclusive and effective across different cultural contexts.

Investing time in training isn't just about adding letters to a name; it's about enhancing skills that translate directly into better patient care. As therapists expand their understanding and capabilities, they become more adept at navigating the complex pathways of trauma healing. This growth ultimately leads to more meaningful and sustained recovery for those they serve.

Remaining curious and open to new learning experiences is what keeps the field of trauma therapy evolving. As therapists pursue these opportunities, they redefine their roles not only as caregivers but as lifelong learners committed to making a profound impact in their community. Each new piece of knowledge gained is a tool that empowers both therapist and patient to reclaim time and mental space, leading towards a more hopeful and resilient future.

Advancements in Trauma Therapy

Trauma therapy has seen significant advancements in recent years, as therapists and researchers continue to deepen their understanding of the complex nature of trauma and refine the methods used to treat it. These advancements are not just tweaks to established practices but often represent paradigm shifts in how therapists approach treatment. As a mental health professional, staying informed about these innovations is crucial to providing the best care possible and to remain effective and empathetic in practice.

One key development in trauma therapy has been the integration of neuroscience into therapeutic practices. Understanding the brain's response to trauma has provided new insights into how memories are processed and stored, and this has influenced how therapies are structured. The use of techniques that leverage our growing knowledge of neuroplasticity—such as mindfulness, Eye Movement Desensitization and Reprocessing (EMDR), and somatic therapies—has become more widespread. These approaches help patients reroute neural pathways, effectively enabling them to change their emotional responses to traumatic memories.

EMDR is particularly noteworthy. Originally developed by Francine Shapiro, this psychotherapy treatment has gained substantial acceptance due to its efficacy in alleviating distress associated with traumatic memories. The process involves guided eye movements that help patients process and integrate traumatic experiences. Its adoption across diverse populations and its scalability in different therapeutic settings illustrate its versatility and effectiveness. It challenges the traditional talk-therapy-only model and presents an alternative for individuals for whom verbal processing is difficult or retraumatizing.

Advancements in trauma therapy also include a heightened awareness of the importance of cultural sensitivity. Therapists are increasingly adapting treatment modalities to fit the cultural contexts and personal identities of their clients. Recognizing that trauma does not occur in a vacuum and that cultural background can significantly influence a person's experience of trauma and treatment reception is becoming more standard practice. This cultural shift in therapy encourages practitioners to engage in continuous learning and self-reflection to better serve diverse populations.

Moreover, trauma-informed care has emerged as a critical advancement in the field. This approach emphasizes understanding, recognizing, and responding to all types of trauma in patient care. It requires practitioners to evaluate how trauma affects individuals' lives and informs therapeutic decision-making. By fostering an environment that prioritizes safety, trustworthiness, and peer support, trauma-informed care aids in mitigating retraumatization during treatment, promoting healing from a holistic perspective.

Technology's role in trauma therapy has also expanded. The incorporation of digital tools and online platforms is transforming how therapy is delivered and accessed. Remote therapy or teletherapy provides flexibility and accessibility for individuals who may have barriers to attending in-person sessions. Additionally, virtual reality (VR) is being explored as a therapeutic tool for immersing patients in safe, controlled environments to process traumatic experiences, providing real-time interactions that can enhance engagement and outcomes.

The integration of mind-body approaches in trauma therapy signifies another vital development. Techniques such as yoga and meditation have gained empirical support as effective adjunctive treatments. These practices emphasize the connection between mental and physical health, encouraging clients to build self-awareness and resilience through nurturing and attuning to their bodily sensations. Practitioners are finding that when combined with other therapeutic interventions, mind-body approaches can accelerate healing and improve overall well-being.

Another significant advancement is the focus on attachment theory and its applications in trauma therapy. Understanding the role of early attachment experiences in shaping how individuals form relationships and process trauma has led to targeted interventions. Therapists are now better equipped to help clients understand and work through dysfunctional attachment patterns shaped by traumatic experiences, leading to healthier relationships and improved mental health.

Continued research and specialization in treating specific trauma populations have also carved new pathways in trauma therapy. For example, specialized approaches have been developed for military veterans, children and adolescents, and survivors of specific types of trauma such as domestic violence or childhood abuse. These targeted therapies employ interventions tailored to the unique challenges and needs presented by different types of trauma.

For mental health professionals, adopting these advancements requires ongoing education and professional development. The landscape of trauma therapy is ever-evolving, and therapists must stay abreast of new research findings and therapeutic techniques. Continuing education workshops, seminars, and online courses offer valuable opportunities to expand knowledge and enhance clinical practice, ultimately improving outcomes for clients.

Lastly, the recognition of therapist well-being as an integral aspect of effective trauma therapy marks an essential advancement. Professionals are encouraged to understand the impact of vicarious trauma and burnout, and to implement self-care strategies to sustain their mental health. This shift not only supports the therapists themselves but also enhances the therapeutic relationship and efficacy of treatment.

In essence, the advancements in trauma therapy reflect a more nuanced and science-informed approach that expands beyond simply addressing symptoms. It embraces a holistic, multifaceted strategy that considers the entire human experience. By keeping pace with these developments, therapists can continue to empower their clients to transform trauma into a journey of healing and resilience.

Building CPT Expertise

Building expertise in Cognitive Processing Therapy (CPT) isn't just about acquiring a set of skills; it's about fostering a mindset of continuous growth and adaptability. As mental health professionals, you're tasked not only with understanding CPT at a fundamental level but also with transforming this understanding into practice that's effective and empathetic. This journey begins with a deep dive into foundational knowledge, but it stretches into the continual honing of skills, responding to new research, and adapting techniques to fit diverse populations and complex cases.

The foundation of CPT expertise lies in mastering its core principles and techniques. This means not only understanding cognitive restructuring and trauma-focused methodologies but also being able to creatively apply these concepts in real-world therapy settings. Whether dealing with a veteran grappling with combat memories or a child coping with early life trauma, the nuances of CPT demand an adaptable yet structured approach. Flexibility within the framework allows therapists to meet patients where they are, offering personalized pathways toward healing.

For those committed to excellence in CPT, a robust understanding of the latest advancements in trauma therapy is essential. Research in the field is ever-evolving, and staying abreast of these changes ensures that your practice remains relevant and effective. This might involve delving into new empirical studies that examine the effectiveness of CPT or exploring innovative therapeutic tools that complement traditional techniques. Staying informed is not merely an academic exercise; it's an ethical obligation to provide the best care possible for those who entrust you with their mental health.

Engagement in professional development is crucial. Participating in workshops, webinars, and certification programs tailored to CPT can enhance your skills and deepen your understanding. These opportunities not only expand your theoretical knowledge but also offer a platform to practice new techniques in a supportive environment. Engaging with colleagues through supervision or peer support groups can provide valuable feedback and new perspectives, fostering a culture of shared learning and growth.

Moreover, mentorship can play a pivotal role in building CPT expertise. For both new and seasoned therapists, seeking out a mentor or serving as one can catalyze professional growth and development. Mentorship allows for the exchange of wisdom and experiences, providing a framework within which complex cases can be dissected and new solutions can be forged. This relational aspect of learning can enrich your practice and offer support during challenging times, ensuring that you're equipped to handle the emotional weight of trauma therapy.

The lens through which we view therapy must also include cultural competence and sensitivity. Building CPT expertise requires an awareness of, and respect for, the diverse backgrounds and experiences of those seeking support. Understanding cultural nuances, societal influences, and individual histories allows for more meaningful and impactful therapy relationships. Culturally responsive care is not just a layer of additional consideration; it is integral to the therapeutic process, ensuring that interventions are relevant, accessible, and effective for all clients.

In addition to individual therapy expertise, group therapy presents another dimension of proficiency within CPT. Facilitating group sessions necessitates a skill set that differs from one-on-one interactions. Group dynamics, collective trauma experiences, and the shared healing journey create a unique environment that requires a different set of interventions and strategies. Building expertise here involves understanding how to harness the power of group support while managing interpersonal dynamics and ensuring all voices are heard and acknowledged.

Another vital area of expertise development in CPT is the ability to integrate technology effectively in the therapy process. Digital tools and teletherapy options have emerged as critical components in reaching a broader client base and overcoming geographical and logistical barriers. Understanding how to incorporate these tools while maintaining ethical standards and ensuring patient privacy adds another layer of complexity to CP, which must be mastered by those aspiring to excellence in the field.

A commitment to quality in CPT also includes evaluating and tailoring treatment plans to ensure optimal patient outcomes continually. Regular monitoring of patient progress, soliciting feedback, and making data- driven adjustments are essential practices. This iterative process is crucial not only for individual client success but also for the ongoing refinement of therapists' skills and approaches.

Finally, developing CPT expertise means addressing personal challenges and practicing self-care. The therapeutic profession is emotionally demanding, and recognizing signs of burnout or vicarious trauma is crucial. Implementing self-care strategies and seeking professional support when needed ensures longevity and sustainability in your practice, allowing you to assist others more effectively over the long term.

Pathways to building CPT expertise are manifold and cumulatively serve to enhance your therapeutic capabilities. By embracing a continuous learning process, practitioners can offer hope and healing to those who need it the most, embodying the kind of transformative and resilient presence that is so desperately needed in the field of trauma therapy today.

CHAPTER 24

FUTURE DIRECTIONS IN TRAUMA THERAPY

As we tentatively step into the future of trauma therapy, we're greeted with an expansive horizon of possibilities that promise to deepen and expand our understanding and effectiveness in healing. Emerging research continues to push boundaries, integrating neuroscience with psychotherapy to unveil new insights into the mechanisms of trauma and recovery.

Innovative therapeutic approaches, such as virtual reality and artificial intelligence, are creating unprecedented opportunities for immersive and personalized treatment experiences. Meanwhile, the growing emphasis on collaboration across disciplines—bringing together psychologists, neuroscientists, and even technologists—suggests a rich, interdisciplinary future for trauma therapy, one that acknowledges and addresses the complexities of human experience. It's a journey driven by empathy and dedication, aiming to reclaim not just the mental space but also the time spent wrestling with past traumas, empowering both patients and practitioners to foster resilience and healing.

Emerging Research

In the ever-evolving field of trauma therapy, emerging research stands as a beacon of hope and innovation. It's an exciting time to explore new methodologies and breakthroughs that have the potential to revolutionize the way we understand and treat trauma. Empirical studies are increasingly shedding light on mechanisms of healing that were once merely speculative or anecdotal. A keen focus is being placed on understanding the nuanced interplay between the brain, body, and emotional responses.

One of the most groundbreaking areas of research involves the integration of neurobiological findings with therapeutic practices. Scientists are delving deeper into how trauma affects the brain's function and structure, particularly areas like the amygdala, hippocampus, and prefrontal cortex. This knowledge is crucial for developing targeted interventions that can address the physiological underpinnings of post-traumatic stress. Understanding these connections may soon lead to highly personalized therapy approaches, where interventions are tailored to the individual's specific neural profile.

Another burgeoning area of study focuses on emotion regulation and its role in trauma recovery. Research is revealing new ways to enhance emotional processing through techniques that foster resilience and cognitive flexibility. Emerging evidence suggests that therapies incorporating mindfulness and body-centered practices can be particularly effective. These approaches empower individuals to reconnect with their bodies, fortify their emotional endurance, and reaffirm their sense of agency.

Moreover, technological advancements are opening new frontiers in trauma therapy. Virtual reality (VR) and artificial intelligence (AI) are being integrated into therapeutic models to enhance engagement and efficacy. VR, for instance, offers immersive environments that help patients safely confront traumatic memories, while AI can support therapists in tailoring interventions based on real-time data.

This fusion of technology and therapy not only enhances accessibility but also provides novel ways to measure patient progress and adjust treatment strategies dynamically.

Precision medicine is another promising avenue in trauma therapy research. By analyzing genetic, environmental, and lifestyle factors, researchers aim to create individualized treatment plans that are more effective and efficient. Studies are ongoing to identify biomarkers that can indicate trauma severity and predict treatment responses. These developments could potentially minimize trial-and-error approaches in therapy, saving time and resources while maximizing therapeutic outcomes.

Cultural competence in trauma therapy is drawing increasing attention in the research community. Scholars are exploring how cultural beliefs and practices impact trauma experiences and healing processes. This research is critical for developing interventions that are not only effective but also culturally sensitive and inclusive. As our communities grow ever more diverse, the ability to provide therapeutically valuable, culturally-aware support becomes indispensable.

On the horizon, we also see promising investigations into alternative and complementary therapies. Treatments like Eye Movement Desensitization and Reprocessing (EMDR), yoga, and acupuncture are being studied for their efficacy in alleviating trauma symptoms. Emerging data is beginning to validate their use, highlighting the potential benefits of integrating such modalities into conventional therapeutic frameworks to enhance overall health and well-being.

Research into the impact of trauma on biological systems, such as the immune and endocrine systems, is gaining momentum as well. Understanding how trauma influences bodily functions can guide us in crafting interventions that address both psychological and physical health. This holistic perspective acknowledges the profound interconnectedness of mind and body in the journey towards healing.

Continued investigation into the role of social support in trauma recovery is vital. Studies are examining how community resources, peer support systems, and family dynamics influence treatment outcomes. By harnessing the power of social connections, therapists can develop strategies that bolster the supportive networks surrounding individuals, reinforcing therapy's impact far beyond the clinical setting.

Finally, the commitment to interprofessional collaboration is driving advancements in trauma therapy research. Bringing together experts from fields such as neuroscience, psychology, social work, and medicine allows for the integration of diverse perspectives and skills. This collaborative approach not only enhances the depth of research but also fosters innovation in developing interventions that are truly comprehensive and effective.

In sum, the landscape of trauma therapy is enriched by a wealth of emerging research. As we continue to discover and validate new therapeutic approaches, the potential to transform trauma treatment becomes more tangible. Equipped with cutting-edge insights and methods, mental health professionals are better prepared to empower individuals to reclaim their lives, fostering resilience and promoting profound healing. This journey is not just about alleviating symptoms, but about facilitating a deeper sense of recovery and wholeness for every person in need.

Innovative Therapeutic Approaches

As the field of trauma therapy continues to evolve, innovative therapeutic approaches are paving new pathways for healing and recovery. These approaches challenge existing paradigms and explore novel techniques that incorporate emerging research and integrate diverse modalities. Such innovation is not just about new techniques, but about rethinking how we understand trauma and its treatment. Opening the door to these approaches means engaging the creativity and resilience of both therapists and clients.

One promising approach is the integration of somatic therapies, which emphasize the essential connection between mind and body in processing trauma. Traditional therapies have often focused on cognitive and emotional aspects without addressing how trauma is stored in the body. Through methods like somatic experiencing, clinicians help clients become more attuned to their physiological responses. This awareness can be a powerful tool, enabling the release of pent-up energy and facilitating a dynamic form of healing that transcends verbal articulation.

Another dimension that is gaining traction is the use of technology in trauma therapy. With advancements in virtual reality (VR) and digital platforms, therapists are exploring new realms of patient engagement. VR, in particular, offers unique opportunities for exposure therapy in controlled environments. It allows patients to confront and process traumatic memories safely, often with greater emotional distance. Additionally, digital tools can enhance accessibility, giving individuals the opportunity to engage in therapy from the comfort and safety of their own space.

Art and creativity-based therapies are also making waves, reminding us that healing can occur through non-traditional means. Art therapy, for instance, offers a way to communicate experiences and emotions that are difficult to verbalize. By tapping into the creative process, individuals can express and reshape their trauma narratives. Music therapy, similarly, uses rhythm and sound to help in emotional regulation and the formation of new, positive associations. These therapies harness creativity as a therapeutic force, thereby offering patients a reinvigorated sense of agency and hope.

Emerging research in neurobiology provides exciting possibilities for therapeutic interventions.

Understanding that trauma can rewire the brain underscores the importance of approaches that promote neuroplasticity. Techniques such as mindfulness and meditation are being woven into therapy protocols to foster present-moment awareness and emotional balance. These practices are shown to contribute to changes in brain structure and function, reinforcing adaptive pathways and softening the grip of traumatic memories.

Peer support models offer another innovative avenue, highlighting the strength of community in recovery. Group settings provide individuals with shared experiences a sense of belonging and validation. This approach emphasizes that healing is not just an individual journey, but a collective one. It leverages the power of shared understanding and the support of empathetic listeners who have walked similar paths.

Furthermore, recent explorations into psychopharmacology and psychedelic-assisted therapy are opening new discussions and avenues in trauma treatment. Substances like MDMA and psilocybin are being studied for their potential to facilitate profound emotional breakthroughs. These substances, when administered in controlled clinical settings, can provide patients with new perspectives and emotional relief, potentially accelerating the therapeutic process.

The innovation doesn't end with new modalities. The evolution of trauma therapy also involves refining existing techniques by integrating new insights and cultural considerations. As treatment becomes more culturally competent, therapists are examining how culture influences trauma and healing. By incorporating cultural sensitivity and adapting practices to meet the unique background of each client, therapists can offer more personalized and effective care.

In embracing these innovative approaches, it's crucial for therapists to remain flexible and open to continuous learning. The landscape of trauma therapy is not static, and adaptability is key in responding to the diverse and evolving needs of clients. Professional development and collaboration across disciplines will drive the advancement of new methodologies and ensure that practitioners are equipped to deliver cutting-edge treatment.

Ultimately, innovative therapeutic approaches aim to empower individuals on their journey to recovery, transforming trauma from a source of suffering into a catalyst for growth and resilience. By integrating these diverse methods, therapists can offer hope and foster healing, enabling clients to reclaim their lives with renewed vitality and purpose.

Collaboration Across Disciplines

The future of trauma therapy lies in the conscious and strategic integration of multidisciplinary approaches. As we recognize the complex interplay of biological, psychological, and social factors in trauma, it's paramount that various disciplines converge to enrich therapeutic outcomes. The adage "it takes a village" rings especially true in trauma therapy, where the diversity of professional perspectives can lead to more holistic and nuanced care.

At the heart of this collaboration is the understanding that no single discipline holds all the answers. Clinical psychologists, psychiatrists, social workers, neuroscientists, medical doctors, and even creative arts therapists can all contribute to a richer, more comprehensive understanding of trauma. By working together, these professionals can break down the silos that often exist in the mental health field, creating a cohesive network that supports the patient from multiple angles.

Imagine a therapy team where a psychiatrist provides medication management, while a social worker addresses environmental stressors. Concurrently, a psychologist delivers evidence-based therapies like Cognitive Processing Therapy (CPT), and a neuroscientist offers insights into brain patterns associated with PTSD. When these elements are coordinated, patients benefit from a treatment plan that acknowledges and addresses the multifaceted nature of their experiences.

Collaboration also means embracing emerging areas of expertise that contribute novel insights to trauma therapy. For instance, the role of nutritionists and exercise physiologists in designing lifestyle interventions that reduce stress and improve overall well-being cannot be underestimated. Engaging occupational therapists can aid in restoring daily functioning, while spiritual counselors might provide comfort and meaning reconstruction for those whose trauma has shaken their faith or core beliefs.

Research is a crucial area where interdisciplinary collaboration can drive the field forward. By pooling their resources and expertise, professionals across disciplines can conduct comprehensive studies that explore the efficacy of integrated therapeutic approaches. These collaborations foster an environment of mutual learning, where each professional's perspective contributes to a more robust understanding of trauma therapy.

Education and training for trauma therapists can also benefit from interdisciplinary collaboration. Cross-disciplinary workshops and seminars can provide therapists with insights beyond their primary focus, equipping them with a broader set of tools and approaches for treatment. Exposure to different modalities can spark creativity and innovation, which are key in adapting to the evolving needs of patients.

The challenge, of course, lies in setting up systems that facilitate these collaborations. There's a need for structures that support shared decision- making, open communication, and respect for the unique perspectives each professional brings. Interdisciplinary teams should foster an environment where all voices are heard and valued, ensuring that no expert overshadows another's contribution.

Technology offers promising avenues to enhance collaboration among disciplines. Digital platforms can serve as a hub for sharing patient information, coordinating care plans, and discussing treatment progress in real-time. Teletherapy and virtual consultations open doors for experts from different geographical locations to collaborate, transcending physical barriers.

As we look towards the future, the mental health landscape calls for a commitment to collaboration that goes beyond mere cooperation. It requires a cultural shift where the sharing of knowledge, resources, and strategies becomes the norm. This collaborative culture can transform how trauma therapy is delivered, making it more dynamic, responsive, and patient-centered.

Ultimately, collaboration across disciplines promotes a sense of community and shared responsibility. It strengthens the commitment of mental health professionals to their patients and emphasizes that we are all working toward a common goal: the healing and empowerment of those who have suffered trauma.

In this interconnected approach, trauma therapy becomes not just a clinical practice but a collective endeavor, striving towards a future where all individuals can reclaim their time and mental space.

CHAPTER
25

ADDRESSING VICARIOUS TRAUMA

Vicarious trauma is an insidious challenge that can affect even the most resilient mental health professionals, quietly seeping into one's psyche through repeated exposure to others' traumatic experiences. Recognizing its signs early is crucial to mitigating its impact, enabling therapists to maintain their empathic engagement without sacrificing personal well- being. As you traverse this fulfilling yet demanding field, embracing robust self-care strategies becomes an imperative act of professional responsibility. Utilizing reflective practices, establishing clear boundaries, and fostering a supportive professional network are not luxuries but necessities. Remember, seeking mentorship or professional support is not a sign of weakness; instead, it's a vital component of enduring in this noble vocation. Empower yourself by prioritizing personal resilience alongside clinical expertise, ensuring a sustainable career that honors both your patients' needs and your mental health. In achieving this balance, you contribute to a healthier life journey for your clients and yourself, modeling the very healing and empowerment you aspire to facilitate.

Vicarious trauma, though often overlooked, can subtly accumulate over time, affecting therapists' ability to provide compassionate care if not addressed proactively. Research has shown that mental health professionals who are frequently exposed to traumatic stories are at risk of experiencing symptoms similar to those of their clients, including emotional numbness, intrusive thoughts, and a diminished sense of hope. Recognizing and understanding vicarious trauma is key to preventing burnout and maintaining therapeutic effectiveness. Regularly engaging in personal reflection, mindfulness, or creative outlets can serve as effective tools for mitigating the emotional toll of this work. Moreover, maintaining professional boundaries is not only vital for preserving mental well-being but also enhances the therapeutic relationship, ensuring that therapists are able to remain present and emotionally available without becoming overwhelmed by the trauma of their clients.

In addition to individual self-care, building a strong, supportive professional network is essential for combating vicarious trauma. Studies show that therapists who engage in peer supervision, team debriefings, or mentorship are better equipped to process the emotional weight of their work and prevent isolation. These spaces allow for the sharing of experiences, the offering of emotional support, and the development of collective coping strategies. By nurturing a sense of camaraderie and mutual care among colleagues, therapists can bolster their emotional resilience while fostering a sense of solidarity in the field. This professional community becomes a vital resource for maintaining emotional balance and sustaining long-term career satisfaction. Ultimately, the ability to model self-care and emotional resilience serves as a powerful example for clients, reinforcing the therapeutic message that healing requires not only dedication to others but also commitment to one's own health and well-being.

Recognizing Signs in Therapists

Vicarious trauma, while rooted in the empathetic and compassionate engagement with clients, manifests uniquely across the spectrum of mental health professionals. It's akin to walking in the emotional shoes of another, sometimes without realizing that those shoes don't fit. Recognizing the signs of vicarious trauma in oneself and others isn't merely beneficial; it's a crucial aspect of sustainable mental health practice. The subtlety and complexity of these signs mean that they might creep in unnoticed, camouflaged by the daily grind and unnoticed demands that accompany the therapist's role.

One of the primary indicators of vicarious trauma is a noticeable shift in a therapist's worldview. When a professional consistently listens to stories of trauma and adversity, it can lead to a pervasive feeling of cynicism or hopelessness about the world. The perspective that the world is inherently unsafe or that people can't be trusted might take root, which starkly contrasts with a therapist's natural inclination towards empathy and understanding. This shift can occur gradually, and therapists are often the last to notice this erosion of their initial idealism.

Emotional exhaustion is another prominent sign, often manifesting as chronic fatigue that leaps beyond typical work-related tiredness. This kind of exhaustion doesn't abate easily with rest. Instead, it lingers, draining enthusiasm and joy from both professional and personal spheres of life. Therapists may find themselves more irritable or overly involved in the emotional distress of others, unable to leave work behind when they close their office doors. This exhaustion places a weight on every conversation, every interaction, affecting the quality of care provided and the therapist's overall well-being.

Physical symptoms may also emerge. These can include headaches, insomnia, and other stress-related ailments. It's essential that therapists pay attention to these bodily cues. Often, our bodies react to stress before our minds have fully processed the emotional load we're carrying. Ignoring these signs can lead to more severe health problems down the line, leaving therapists incapacitated and unable to perform their duties at all.

Therapists might also notice changes in their emotional responses. Feeling detached from clients, emotionally numb, or experiencing unusually heightened emotions such as anger and sadness could be red flags. These symptoms point to an internal overload where the mind and body are struggling to process the emotional barrage they are experiencing. It's like a sponge reaching its saturation point—there's simply no more room to absorb.

Professional relationships with clients can be affected as well. A therapist might find themselves developing uncharacteristic impatience or irritability towards those in their care. Alternatively, there might be an over-identification with clients' problems, leading to blurred boundaries. These changes can compromise the effectiveness of therapy, as trust between therapist and client erodes. The therapeutic alliance, which is foundational to successful outcomes, becomes strained.

A decline in professional performance is also a clear sign. Missed deadlines, reduced concentration, lack of enthusiasm for professional development, and a general disengagement from workplace activities can indicate that vicarious trauma is taking its toll. These are often overlooked as they can be misattributed to temporary stress or workload issues, yet they offer valuable insights into the underlying impact of vicarious trauma.

Social withdrawal is another symptom, often mystifying to those around the affected individual. Therapists accustomed to engaging deeply with others may begin to isolate themselves. Social activities that once offered enjoyment or relaxation turn into burdens, exacerbating the sense of disconnection and loneliness. Recognizing this withdrawal and its impact on personal relationships can be pivotal in addressing the cascading effects of vicarious trauma.

Finally, a pervasive sense of inefficacy can besiege therapists. This feeling can stem from a sense of stagnation in client progress or an unfounded belief that they're not doing enough, despite evidence to the contrary. This erosion of professional self-efficacy is often compounded by the intrinsic value therapists place on making a positive difference in their clients' lives. A shift in confidence and capability can lead to a crisis in professional identity, triggering further emotional distress.

It's crucial for therapists to routinely engage in self-reflection and self- assessment. Setting aside time to truly check in with oneself, away from the demands of client sessions and administrative responsibilities, can prevent the insidious onset of vicarious trauma. Therapeutic supervision and peer support are invaluable tools for maintaining this awareness. When therapists can openly discuss their experiences and feelings without fear of judgment, they create a pathway to recognition and management of vicarious trauma.

Organizational supports play a significant role in recognizing and mitigating these signs. Workplaces that prioritize therapist well-being often incorporate regular training sessions on vicarious trauma and its signs. Such proactive measures arm therapists with the resources and knowledge they need to protect their mental health and sustain their practice over the long term.

In essence, recognizing the signs of vicarious trauma isn't just about identifying problems—it's about taking the first step towards healing. Therapists, equipped with self-awareness and supported by their professional networks, can address these symptoms robustly, ensuring they remain effective, compassionate, and fulfilled in their roles. The journey of a therapist is one of profound impact; sustaining this journey requires vigilance in self-care and a commitment to noticing when the scales tip from health to harm.

Implementing Self-Care Strategies

In the intricate dance of trauma therapy, practitioners serve as both guides and vessels. They bear witness to stories etched with deep pain, and while their professional armor might appear impenetrable, it's crucial to acknowledge the porous nature of empathy. Vicarious trauma is not an isolated affliction reserved for a few; it subtly permeates the lives of even the most seasoned mental health professionals. That's why self-care isn't merely an option; it's an imperative.

Implementing self-care strategies begins with the fundamental understanding that it's not about luxury, but necessity. Imagine a vessel carefully crafted to contain the myriad stories of healing and hardship. Without regular maintenance, this vessel might crack under pressure, its capability to safeguard and support compromised. For therapists, regular self-care is the necessary maintenance that ensures their vessel remains intact and can continue holding space for others.

In practice, self-care strategies must be as individualized as the therapy itself. One universal truth, however, is the significance of establishing boundaries. Boundaries serve as a crucial buffer, allowing mental health professionals to delineate between their personal and professional worlds. This separation is essential for leaving work at work, something as simple as not checking emails or client updates during personal time. Establishing clear start and end times for workday ensures that free time is truly restorative.

Another cornerstone of effective self-care is engaging in regular physical activity. Movement counteracts the sedentary nature of clinical work, permitting the release of built-up tension. Whether it's a brisk walk, yoga, or a spirited dance class, movement helps disperse the emotional load carried after a day of client sessions. Physical activity isn't just about bodily health; it's a mental cleanse, a recalibration that primes therapists to be fully present in their next interaction.

Beyond the physical, emotional nourishment is vital. This can mean participating in activities that bring joy and relaxation: hobbies, spending time with loved ones, or engaging in creative pursuits. Therapists often recommend such strategies to their clients, but it's equally important they 'walk the talk'. Engaging in fulfilling activities serves as both a reminder of their humanity and a confirmation that life is rich and multi- dimensional, extending beyond the boundaries of their clinical roles.

Maintaining a supportive professional network is another strategic pillar. Peer groups or supervision sessions offer a safe harbor where clinicians can navigate the turbulent waters of challenging cases and complex emotions. Discussing cases with peers helps distribute the emotional load, offering fresh perspectives and insights. It fosters a sense of not being alone in the healing journey, reaffirming that shared experiences create a buffer against the weight of vicarious trauma.

Mental health professionals also benefit from cultivating mindfulness practices. Mindfulness teaches present awareness, an antidote to the emotionally taxing nature of dwelling in the traumas of others. For some, mindfulness may manifest in meditation or breathwork, for others, through mindful eating or walking. What matters is the underlying principle: staying grounded in the present, thereby providing an emotional anchor amidst the tide of other people's stories.

Just as intake assessments are critical in understanding a client's needs, periodic self-check-ins are essential for therapists to gauge their emotional and mental well-being. These check-ins could involve journaling, attending personal therapy, or simply reflecting on one's energy levels and emotional state. Being honest with oneself about the signs of fatigue or stress ensures that preventive actions are taken before burnout ensues.

Nutrition and sleep also play integral roles in maintaining therapists' resiliency. Eating balanced meals and prioritizing good sleep hygiene can profoundly impact a professional's daily performance and emotional state. Proper nutrition fuels the body, bolstering focus and mood, while adequate rest provides the recovery needed to tackle another day's challenges positively.

In scenarios where self-care strategies seem inadequate, seeking professional support is vital. Therapists are not immune to needing therapy themselves. Engaging in therapy offers a structured opportunity to process emotions and gain insights that can propel personal and professional growth. This practice models strength in vulnerability and reinforces the idea that everyone can benefit from professional guidance, regardless of their expertise in the field.

In conclusion, self-care is not an afterthought but a foundational aspect of sustaining a fruitful career in mental health. It ensures that therapists remain capable of compassionate care, providing a nurturing sanctuary for clients navigating the stormy seas of trauma. As healers investing in their well-being, they honor both their professional journey and their personal lives, creating a harmonious balance that allows them to thrive, not just survive. The path of self-care is ongoing, demanding intentional choices and continual reflection, yet it's the key to unlocking long-term resilience and fulfillment in both the personal and professional realms.

Seeking Professional Support

In the field of trauma therapy, clinicians and mental health professionals are constantly exposed to the emotional burdens of their clients. This repeated exposure, although a testament to their dedication, can often lead to what is known as vicarious trauma. Recognizing one's limits and seeking professional support is not just beneficial—it's essential to maintain personal well-being and continue providing effective care.

The first step is acknowledging that needing support doesn't equate to weakness or inadequacy. In fact, it's a vital aspect of self-awareness and professional growth. By seeking help, therapists not only protect themselves but also model healthy practices for their clients. It's about fostering a balanced view of strength that combines vulnerability with resilience.

Professional supervision is a cornerstone in managing vicarious trauma. Supervision offers a structured environment where therapists can relate their experiences without judgment. It becomes a safe harbor for discussing difficult cases, sharing emotional reactions, and receiving guidance. Through these interactions, therapists can gain fresh perspectives that not only aid in personal coping but also enhance therapeutic approaches.

Collegial support groups provide another valuable resource. Such groups serve as communal spaces where professionals with similar experiences can gather to share, listen, and learn from one another. The collective wisdom of the group can be empowering, transforming experiences of isolation into moments of connection and shared understanding.

In addition to supervision and peer groups, engaging in ongoing professional education and training can help therapists develop effective strategies to handle vicarious trauma. Understanding the latest research and techniques offers new tools for dealing with both personal and clinical challenges. It also keeps therapy practices up to date, making them more adaptable to the diverse needs of clients.

Many therapists also find it beneficial to work with their own therapist or counselor. This personal therapeutic relationship allows for the exploration of deeper emotional responses and issues that may arise from their professional work. By engaging in therapy, mental health professionals can experience firsthand the therapeutic processes they provide to their clients, which can deepen empathy and enrich their practice.

It's crucial for healthcare providers to establish work-life boundaries to ensure that their professional duties do not overwhelm their personal lives. Setting specific times for client interactions, adhering to work schedules, and disconnecting after hours are practical steps. These measures help prevent burnout and maintain mental health outside of the clinical setting.

Another aspect of professional support is self-reflection and mindfulness practices. Being mindful allows therapists to remain grounded and attentive to their personal experiences of stress and anxiety. Techniques such as meditation, journaling, and other reflective practices can be powerful tools in building resilience against the effects of vicarious trauma.

Employers and professional organizations can play a significant role in providing resources and creating environments conducive to the mental health of therapists. Policies that promote mental well-being, such as reasonable caseloads, regular breaks, and access to mental health services, can make a substantial difference. A supportive workplace culture encourages professionals to seek help proactively and without fear of stigma.

Ultimately, seeking professional support is about creating a sustainable career in trauma care. Therapists committed to their own health and well-being demonstrate a compassionate approach to the very principles they teach. They become beacons for their clients—showing that asking for help is not just okay, but exemplary.

In this journey of offering healing and hope, it is vital to remember that well-supported therapists are better poised to deliver effective and empathetic care. By prioritizing professional support, therapists can navigate the challenges of their work with grace and preserve their passion and commitment to serving others.

CONCLUSION

As we stand at the precipice of our exploration into Cognitive Processing Therapy (CPT) and its profound influence on addressing post-traumatic stress disorder (PTSD), it is essential to pause and reflect on the journey we've undertaken. This book has sought to unravel the complexities of trauma therapy, equipping you with a treasure trove of knowledge and practical strategies to empower not only your practice but also your personal growth as a healthcare provider. Through this, we aim to reclaim time and mental space—a feat that is as rewarding as it is challenging.

The heart of trauma therapy rests on the delicate yet powerful dynamic of the therapeutic alliance. In establishing trust with your patients, you not only foster an environment conducive to healing but also give them space to explore their narratives safely. This relationship is not just about offering solutions; it's about being a witness to their stories, validating their experiences, and guiding them gently toward self-discovery and healing.

Armed with the core principles of CPT, we have traversed the nuances of cognitive restructuring, learning how to recognize and challenge maladaptive thoughts that keep our clients bound to their traumatic pasts. The journey to recovery is not linear, nor is it uniform. Every patient presents a unique tapestry of experiences, beliefs, and emotions that must be woven thoughtfully into the therapeutic process. Remember, your role as a therapist is to serve as both a guide and a collaborator in this intricate process.

We've also shone a light on the importance of cultural sensitivity and the necessity of adapting therapeutic techniques to resonate with diverse populations. By appreciating the various lenses through which patients view their experiences, you become more equipped to offer personalized care that honors their cultural backgrounds and individual preferences.

Adapting CPT to meet these needs is not merely about addressing differences; it's about amplifying our understanding and fostering inclusivity within mental health care.

In addressing the special considerations for populations such as veterans, children, and those with co-occurring disorders, we've underscored the need for therapists to be attuned to both the particular traumas and the broader contexts affecting these groups. This attentiveness enriches the therapeutic process and enhances the chances of successful outcomes.

We must also recognize the resilience and, at times, the vulnerability of providers themselves. Working intimately with trauma can inevitably lead to vicarious trauma, which underscores the importance of self-care and professional support. Balancing empathy with preservation of personal well-being is crucial in sustaining a long and fruitful career in trauma therapy.

Looking to the future, the landscape of trauma therapy is ever-evolving. Technological advancements offer new modalities for therapy yet pose ethical implications that require careful consideration. Staying abreast of emerging research and innovative approaches will empower you to integrate these advancements into your practice effectively.

Ultimately, the foundation of all therapeutic practice resides in ongoing education and collaboration. As new research and methodologies emerge, continuous learning ensures that your skills remain sharp and relevant.

Seek out training opportunities, engage with your peers across disciplines, and remain open to novel therapeutic strategies.

By understanding, adapting, and embracing the wealth of knowledge and strategies available, you are uniquely positioned to empower both yourself and those you serve. The journey you've embarked upon with this book is but the beginning of a lifelong commitment to growth, understanding, and healing. Together, we can foster a world where recovery is not just an aspiration but a reality for all who seek it.

APPENDIX A

APPENDIX

In this appendix, you'll find a collection of resources, case studies, and practical tools designed to aid you on your journey to empower both yourself and those you serve. The additional resources include recommended readings, evidence-based articles, and online platforms that expand on practices highlighted throughout the book. Case studies provide illustrative examples of diverse trauma scenarios and their nuanced approaches, offering insights into real-world application. You'll also find worksheets and handouts that are integral to reinforcing the cognitive processing therapy (CPT) techniques discussed. Designed for seamless integration into your practice, these materials aim to support your personal and professional growth, helping you reclaim your time and mental space while providing exceptional care. Embrace this appendix as a companion in your ongoing commitment to healing and resilience, much like a toolkit crafted to meet the unique challenges faced by healthcare providers, researchers, clinical supervisors, educators, graduate students, trainees, and mental health professionals navigating the complex landscape of mental health care.

Additional Resources

As you navigate the complex and ever-evolving field of trauma therapy, access to a variety of resources can empower and enhance your practice. The significance of staying informed and supported in this work can't be overstated, and this section aims to guide you toward valuable materials and platforms to bolster your journey. From academic journals to online forums, each resource serves as a stepping stone in the continuous path of learning and personal growth.

One of the primary resources available to mental health professionals is scholarly journals. Publications like the *Journal of Traumatic Stress* and *Psychological Trauma: Theory, Research, Practice, and Policy* offer peer- reviewed articles that delve into the latest research findings. These journals present evidence-based practices and innovative approaches that are instrumental for professionals dedicated to staying abreast of new developments in trauma therapy.

Beyond academic journals, books written by leading figures in trauma therapy provide comprehensive insights that can enhance therapeutic practice. Works by pioneers in the field often combine empirical research with poignant case studies, offering both theoretical and practical insights. Titles that focus specifically on Cognitive Processing Therapy (CPT) and Post-Traumatic Stress Disorder (PTSD) are invaluable for experts aiming to deepen their understanding and application of these concepts.

Online platforms and communities also play a crucial role in connecting professionals. Websites like Trauma-Focused Cognitive Behavioral Therapy (TF-CBT) provide valuable resources, including training modules and instructional videos. These sites often host forums where practitioners can share experiences, discuss challenges, and provide mutual support. By engaging with such communities, mental health professionals can overcome the isolation that often accompanies the therapeutic profession.

Professional organizations offer another layer of support and information. Associations such as the International Society for Traumatic Stress Studies (ISTSS) or the American Psychological Association (APA) often host annual conferences, webinars, and workshops. These events are prime opportunities to network, share findings, and learn from leaders in the field. Attending these gatherings not only enhances one's expertise but also provides needed inspiration and motivation.

Conferences and symposiums dedicated to trauma therapy allow practitioners to immerse themselves in emerging trends and novel approaches. These events frequently include presentations on cutting-edge research, roundtable discussions with experts, and training sessions in therapeutic strategies. Attendees often leave these gatherings with refreshed perspectives and enhanced skills, ready to apply this new knowledge in their practices.

Digital tools, such as mobile apps and software designed for psychological support, have become increasingly significant in the practice of trauma therapy. Apps designed to facilitate patient engagement, track therapy progress, or offer psychoeducation can be seamlessly integrated into treatment plans. These tools also empower patients to take an active role in their healing process, providing them with resources to manage symptoms outside of therapy sessions.

For those seeking mentorship and individualized guidance, supervision remains a cornerstone in the development of therapeutic expertise.

Supervision offers a safe space to discuss complex cases and receive constructive feedback. By engaging in regular supervision, mental health professionals can refine their techniques, address countertransference issues, and ensure they provide the highest quality of care to their clients.

To support ongoing education, numerous universities and institutions offer specialized courses and certification programs in trauma therapy. These educational opportunities are tailored to various professional levels, from introductory courses for new therapists to advanced certifications focusing on specific modalities. Participation in these programs can lead to professional growth and recognition, heightening one's ability to impact lives positively.

Finally, fostering self-care and well-being as a professional in the mental health field is not only beneficial but essential. Resources dedicated to therapist self-care, such as self-guided therapeutic exercises, yoga classes, mindfulness workshops, and meditation retreats, are vital. They support mental health professionals in maintaining their resilience and passion for the work, preventing burnout, and preserving their capacity to care for others.

In conclusion, the journey to mastery in trauma therapy is ongoing and multifaceted. By utilizing a combination of academic resources, professional communities, digital tools, and self-care strategies, health care providers, researchers, clinical supervisors, educators, graduate students, trainees, and mental health professionals can continue to grow and innovate in their practice. The culmination of these efforts ensures not only the enrichment of their professional lives but also the successful empowerment of their clients on their paths to recovery.

Case Studies and Examples

To truly grasp the transformative power of Cognitive Processing Therapy (CPT) in treating PTSD, real-world case studies provide invaluable insights. Through these narratives, we see the application of CPT principles, its challenges, and the profound benefits it can offer. Each example serves as a testament to the therapeutic journey, illustrating the myriad of experiences encountered by both therapists and patients.

Consider the case of Sarah, a nurse and single mother who had been grappling with PTSD following a traumatic event during a routine hospital shift. Sarah started blaming herself for not being able to prevent the incident, a common cognitive distortion among those with PTSD. Through CPT, she began to unravel these maladaptive belief patterns. Her therapist employed cognitive restructuring techniques, encouraging her to challenge these self-defeating thoughts. Over time, Sarah learned to reframe her beliefs, acknowledging that the incident was beyond her control. This cognitive shift was pivotal in diminishing her symptoms and reclaiming her mental space.

In another case, we have Mark, a veteran struggling with intrusive thoughts and hypervigilance. Mark's initial attachment to his military identity made therapy challenging. However, his therapist incorporated cultural sensitivity into their sessions, creating a safe space where Mark felt understood. This consideration of Mark's unique background allowed for the successful adaptation of CPT techniques to address his needs. By engaging through expressive trauma narratives and challenging core beliefs connected to his military experience, Mark was able to identify the roots of his trauma and work towards healing.

Working with children presents its own set of challenges, as seen in the case of 10-year-old Emma, who experienced a traumatic incident at school. Traditional therapy methods proved less effective due to her developmental stage. Instead, her therapist crafted sessions involving play therapy elements, adapted specifically for her age group. These sessions engaged Emma in a comfortable manner, facilitating emotional recognition and cognitive restructuring. Over time, Emma became more expressive about her feelings, gradually disassociating those from her trauma. This customized approach demonstrates how CPT can be effectively tailored for younger populations.

An intriguing example comes from a group therapy setting, where diverse participants collaborated to dismantle common misconceptions about PTSD. Through structured group sessions, participants like Linda and Jake shared their stories, learning from each other's experiences. This dynamic facilitated mutual support and encouraged self-reflection in ways individual therapy sometimes could not. By observing others challenge their distorted beliefs, participants felt motivated to do the same, creating a synergistic healing environment.

Moreover, the integration of technology has opened new avenues in CPT, as demonstrated by James, who couldn't attend in-person sessions due to geographical and mobility constraints. Through teletherapy, James maintained consistent contact with his therapist, utilizing digital tools like virtual thought records and cognitive restructuring apps. These technologies became part of his therapeutic arsenal, making his treatment both accessible and effective.

An exemplary case involves Anna, a trauma survivor who faced barriers in accessing therapy due to her remote location. Her journey reflects the synergistic power of combining teletherapy with traditional methods.

Through digital tools, Anna stayed connected with her therapist, working through therapy sessions despite the distance. This accessibility was pivotal in helping her maintain therapeutic momentum and overcome logistical barriers, highlighting the potential of integrating technology in CPT.

Then there's the poignant story of Tom, a first responder plagued by recurrent nightmares and avoidance behaviors. His narrative focused therapy sessions involved writing detailed trauma accounts, gradually reducing avoidance and desensitizing Tom to traumatic memories. By iterating through his trauma narrative, Tom found new perspectives, reducing the emotional burden of his memories. This process underscores the effectiveness of therapeutic writing and reading as tools for emotional processing.

For many, integrating CPT into their lives involves not just cognitive changes but also environmental and relational shifts. Clara, a survivor of domestic abuse, exemplified this holistic transformation. As she progressed in therapy, Clara didn't only work on individual belief restructuring but also employed safety planning strategies to ensure her environment aligned with her therapeutic goals. This combination of cognitive and practical approaches provided a comprehensive framework for sustained recovery.

In these varied examples, the adaptability of CPT becomes evident. Whether addressing cultural sensitivities, developmental stages, or logistical challenges, CPT's principles serve as a foundation upon which therapies can be tailored to fit individual needs. The adaptability of the therapy ensures that each patient, regardless of background or circumstance, can work towards reclaiming their mental health and well- being.

What emerges from these stories is a tapestry of human resilience, a powerful reminder of the impact that thoughtful and empathetic therapeutic practice can have. As therapists navigate the complexities of trauma with their patients, these case studies reinforce the importance of continuing education and remaining open to innovative therapeutic approaches. By drawing on both traditional and emerging practices, CPT can be effectively utilized to transform lives, helping individuals across diverse settings to overcome the shackles of their trauma and emerge stronger than ever.

Morksheets and Handouts

In the realm of trauma therapy, particularly Cognitive Processing Therapy (CPT), worksheets and handouts act as indispensable tools that guide both clinicians and clients through the maze of recovery. They aren't just pieces of paper filled with exercises; rather, they're bridges connecting theory to practical application. While the primary focus remains on helping clients internalize therapeutic concepts, these materials also serve to foster self-reflection and deepen understanding.

For healthcare providers, educators, and students, worksheets in a CPT context are meticulously crafted to facilitate structured thought. They offer a blueprint for translating abstract cognitive theories into tangible steps. Each worksheet is a small beacon, illuminating the path from recognizing maladaptive thoughts to developing healthier cognition. In essence, they transform complex cognitive theories into digestible, actionable tasks that can be easily employed in both individual and group settings.

Constructing these worksheets requires an empathetic understanding of the varied experiences that clients bring into therapy. The exercises must be adaptable to culturally diverse populations and mindful of individual predicaments. This not only helps retain a personal touch but also ensures inclusivity, allowing a broader range of clients to benefit from the potential healing that CPT provides. Worksheets aren't static; they're dynamic documents that can be tailored to meet unique therapeutic needs, especially when dealing with populations such as veterans or adolescents.

One of the key elements in these worksheets is their role in challenging and restructuring thoughts. By putting pen to paper, clients can articulate their thought patterns, critically evaluate them, and subsequently work to reshape those that are not serving their recovery. This process inherently empowers clients, granting them the agency to confront and modify maladaptive beliefs. It's an invitation to transform the narrative of trauma into one of resilience and hope.

Handouts, much like worksheets, provide foundational knowledge and practical tips that can be revisited outside the confines of the therapy session. They are instrumental in reinforcing psychoeducation. Whether it's a guide to understanding the neurobiological impacts of trauma or a step-by-step outline for managing intense emotions, handouts serve to contextualize and consolidate learning. They act as a reference point for clients, helping them to consistently engage with therapeutic concepts even beyond the therapeutic hour.

Moreover, handouts offer a form of continuity. In between sessions, they maintain the momentum of therapy, ensuring that the process doesn't lose traction. This is particularly crucial for clients who may struggle with consistency or who face barriers to attending regular sessions. By providing these tangible resources, therapy becomes accessible no matter the setting, empowering clients to take charge of their mental health journey.

For mental health professionals, these tools are more than just aids; they are extensions of therapeutic expertise. They establish a rhythm in therapy sessions, allowing clinicians to map out therapeutic progression with clarity and purpose. Furthermore, they can serve as a catalyst for discussion, prompting clients to voice concerns or insights that may have otherwise remained unspoken. This can lead to breakthroughs that might not be otherwise achieved through dialogue alone.

It's important for therapists to approach these documents with a degree of flexibility. They aren't scripts to be followed rigidly but rather guides that should be adapted to fit the contours of each client's experience. Implementing worksheets and handouts with creativity and sensitivity can enhance their effectiveness, ensuring that therapy resonates deeply on a personal level.

In clinical supervision and education, these tools are invaluable. They provide a practical framework for graduate students and trainees to understand the application of CPT principles. As emerging practitioners familiarize themselves with these worksheets and handouts, they gain insights into the intricacies of therapy dynamics and the importance of patient-centered care. This fosters a holistic understanding of trauma therapy and prepares professionals to devise effective interventions in real-world settings.

Lastly, it's worth acknowledging that these instruments help cultivate a culture of continual learning and adaptation. As therapy evolves, so too must the resources we employ. Feedback from clients and observations from ongoing research continually inform the development of new worksheets and handouts. This iterative process ensures that therapy remains aligned with the best practices and innovatively responsive to the ever-changing landscape of mental health care.

In conclusion, worksheets and handouts are not mere therapeutic supplements; they are fundamental components of the healing process. Through structured reflection and educational reinforcement, they create pathways for growth and understanding that support both clients and professionals in navigating the complexities of trauma recovery. With these tools in hand, the journey towards reclaiming time and mental space becomes not just a feasible endeavor but an inspiring one.